Orthopaedic Medicine
Cyriax
Updated Value in Daily Practice

Part II:
Treatment by Deep Transverse Massage,
Mobilization, Manipulation and Traction

Steven L.H. De Coninck

Published and Distributed by:
OPTP
P.O. Box 47009
Minneapolis, MN 55447-0009
www.OPTP.com

Printed in the U.S.A

Table of Contents

Table of Contents

Chapter 12: Cervical Manipulation and Deep Friction

Acknowledgments

I am amazed at how many people are involved, directly and indirectly, in the development of these books and related video productions. It started, of course, with Dr. Cyriax's life work. The value of and the passion for orthopaedic medicine remains my basic inspiration.

My parents have played a vital role in my personal and professional development with years of continuous love and support. My father, Bob De Coninck, in particular, has been an exemplary role model, since he too has spent many years spreading the knowledge and inspiring colleagues in Cyriax methodology. While participating in updating OMCyriax and the structure of the Cyriax continuing education courses, he continues to pass his passion on to me.

I couldn't imagine that OMCyriax would also have such a profound influence on my private life as well. While teaching a course in Brazil, I met my lovely wife Luciane. Over time, our professional relationship as Cyriax-based colleagues blossomed into the loving relationship that it is today. As my wife and colleague, Luciane keeps me grounded, and she willingly bears the sacrifices our careers occasionally require.

I would like to express my sincere gratitude to all who have given me a chance to follow my passion. I would like to thank Mrs. Shari Schroeder of Orthopaedic Physical Therapy Products for believing in what I do and making these publications possible; to Mr. Frans Cesar, CEO of Gymna, for continually having faith in me and who can always be relied on for extensive professional and logistic support during the recording of new videos and photo shooting.

Claude D'Heedene did a great job again as our film director.

To Maurizio Leone, many thanks for coming to Belgium, especially for the photo shooting.

Thanks to our colleague Ruben Coutteau: he is a great model.

I would like to extend special thanks to Ken Learman, M.Ed., PT, OCS, COMT. Your contribution to the revision of my text was indispensable. Barbara Field and Corry Walbridge expended a lot of effort giving the books the look they deserve.

And last, but certainly not least, thanks to the many colleagues who attend our courses and inspire me to constantly improve.

Introduction

In daily practice, we are regularly confronted with problems related to diagnosis and treatment of soft tissue lesions of the locomotor system. During his career, Dr. Cyriax developed a marvelous diagnostic system based entirely on anatomical logic. History, inspection, functional examination, and, if necessary, palpation and/or diagnostic injection allow the clinician to reach a useful diagnosis in an effective and efficient way. The basic treatment strategy consisting of deep transverse friction massage, manipulation, mobilization, traction, infiltration, or injection prove to be efficient and are very compatible with other techniques as well.

These books are not just about the execution of techniques, but discuss in detail how to detect optimal circumstances for application of techniques. Achieving a useful diagnosis in a safe manner is of primary importance.

Cyriax is perhaps one of the best-known names in the field of orthopaedic medicine, but can we assume that the content behind the name is fully understood as well?

Many people are familiar with some Cyriax philosophical "highlights," but highlights alone, without thorough knowledge of the many important details, leads to inefficiency and an inaccurate image of OMCyriax. Indeed, updated OMCyriax is perhaps even more practical than it has been in the past. It has been said that it forms the basis for many other methods, including McKenzie, Maitland, and Kaltenborn, to name a few, but we have to realize that this basis evolves.

Many Cyriax or Cyriax-related works have already been published. What are the purpose of these new books?

I would like to familiarize the reader with the real value of updated OMCyriax: some views have been abandoned, many others have been confirmed by research. Some practical procedures have been optimized or have become more patient and therapist friendly. The new standardized Cyriax Assessment Forms are also incorporated in the text. Our continuing education courses are based on these new publications. In addition, we offer two new video productions (DVD or VHS) covering all examination and treatment techniques within the OMCyriax field.

I deliberately eschewed producing yet another "scientific" book containing an extensive literature overview, with a plethora of theoretical considerations/references on the biomechanical, histological, and physiological fields. Other very good texts have already covered this material extensively.

My purpose is to offer the reader a truly practical guide for daily use. Your goal is to reach a diagnosis quickly, safely, and effectively; therefore, these references help you decide which questions to ask and why? What are the diagnostic consequences of these questions? How to assess and detect possible alarm signs? How to perform a functional examination and make a differential diagnosis? How to create a treatment strategy and interpret the expectation pattern?

To achieve those goals, I preferred to divide these publications into three parts:

- Part I: Functional Examination and Diagnosis

- Part II: Treatment Using Deep Transverse Friction, Manipulation, Mobilization, and Traction

- Part III: Treatment Using Infiltration and Injection

By truly understanding this updated basis, the link to other methods and some symbiotic compatibility become obvious. There is no need for tunnel vision. It is my sincere conviction that knowing the Cyriax philosophy is an absolute basis for every soft tissue therapist, but it doesn't open all doors; links to other methods are useful and necessary, and vice versa.

"Flying above the clouds,
where the sun is always shining, is nice;
but flying without knowing how to run makes
the landing very painful"

Steven L.H. De Coninck
October 2003

Acronyms

A = active

ADL = activities of daily living

ACL = anterior cruciate ligament

AP = anteroposterior

DD = differential diagnosis

DF = deep transverse massage/friction

FAP = full articular pattern

i.a. = intra-articular

ID = internal derangment

LCL = lateral collateral ligament

MCL = medial collateral ligament

MRI = magnetic resonance imaging

MTJ = musculotendinous junction

NMRI = nuclear magnetic resonance imaging

P = passive

PA = painful arc

PCL = posterior cruciate ligament

PLL = posterior longitudinal ligament

PPLP = primary posterolateral protrusion

R = resisted

RA = rheumatoid arthritis

RP = referred pain

ROM = range of motion

SAIS (ASIS) = anterior superior iliac spine

SLR = straight-leg raise

SPIS = superior posterior iliac spine

ULTT = upper limb tension test

I. General Remarks

Rest is not recommended as a treatment procedure. In acute cases, during the inflammatory phase, the RICE principle (Rest, Ice, Compression, Elevation) is useful. A maximum of 5 days' rest (not longer) is also advisable.

In certain cases, healing without sufficient movement at the site of the lesion leads to imperfect repair and remodeling. Adhesions are created with a chaotic scar ("cross links") and residual symptoms as a result.

The post-traumatic inflammatory reaction also limits mobility at the site of the lesion. Consequently, we should abate it as much as possible, perhaps with deep friction or with triamcinolone infiltration, depending on the site of the lesion.

Some lesions can become self-perpetuating for months or even years, whereas a single infiltration of triamcinolone would suffice to abolish the inflammation, allowing us to restart active treatment and to make the symptoms disappear.

II. Minor Muscular Tears

A muscle must contract; on contraction, it broadens. After an injury, a muscle's ability to broaden may be limited by microscopic adhesions in the muscle. The treatment of a muscular tear must aim at maintaining or restoring the ability to broaden. In a later stage of treatment, we also have to focus on the longitudinal loading of the structure. That is why, in most cases, deep transverse friction will be a good treatment: to move the muscle fibers transversely between themselves, without a longitudinal component (during the first weeks), so as to maintain their normal ability to broaden to prevent or eliminate microscopic adhesions in the muscle.

For three large muscle groups, namely, the quadriceps, hamstrings, and calf muscles, the principles of treatment are slightly different:

- Acute stage:
  - Infiltration of a local anesthetic to reduce the muscle spasm.
  - Deep friction plus active and electrical contractions to optimize the contraction capacity.
- Chronic stage: deep friction plus active and electrical contractions.

For a lesion of any musculotendinous junction throughout the body, the treatment is deep friction and not infiltration.

III. Tendinous Lesions

A. Tendinitis, Tendinosis

The lesions often lie at the tenoperiosteal junction and less often in the body of the tendon. Many of these lesions are of the "self-perpetuating inflammation" type.

Two main treatments must be considered:

- Infiltration of triamcinolone: offers quick results but a rather high rate of recurrence (which is logical since the corticoid doesn't influence scar formation).
- Deep friction: takes more time (average of 3-4 weeks), but there are fewer recurrences.

In the case of tendinosis (i.e., a chronic lesion without the presence of inflammatory cells), the treatment is commenced by deep friction to trigger the healing process. In a later stage, deep friction can be combined with longitudinal stress exercise to optimize the loading capacity of the healing structure.

B. Tenosynovitis, Tenovaginitis

Infiltration with triamcinolone is the first option; if the lesion is too large, deep friction can be considered.

So far, we have only discussed muscular and tendinous lesions. In both cases, another element of treatment should not be neglected: a muscle and a tendon need relative rest during the first weeks and must be spared heavy activity. This is an essential part of the treatment. The patient can also perform a specific home exercise program to further improve the remodeling of the scar tissue.

IV. Minor Ligamentous Sprains

A general principle that is paramount here is that mobilization gets the better of immobilization.

A. Acute Sprain

To reduce the post-traumatic inflammation, use deep friction or triamcinolone (follow RICE for the first 5 days).

To prevent the formation of adhesions, use deep friction and progressive mobilization.

For an acute lesion of the medial collateral ligament at the knee and the lateral ankle ligaments (anterior talofibular, calcaneocuboid, and calcaneofibular ligaments), we proceed as follows:

- Progressive deep friction: 30 seconds ⇒ 3 minutes ⇒ 5 minutes ⇒ 7 minutes ⇒ 10 minutes per session (we need to be very gentle in the acute phase so as not to make the condition worse).

- Progressive mobilization, without causing any pain.

- Marching/proprioceptive exercise.

B. Chronic Sprain

Under the analgesic influence of the deep friction, adhesions are ruptured by manipulation; the patient maintains the new range of movement by incorporating a home exercise program.

V. Exercises?

As described above, the main treatment always includes movement as well in an acute or a chronic lesion. With acute lesions, we have to be careful not to move too much in the first 5 days. With chronic lesions, it is possible during the first days of treatment to provoke an increase of symptoms. This is a normal reaction for a chronic lesion that has not healed appropriately; the healing mechanism is triggered again.

The therapist provides specific movement by using deep friction. This happens an average of three to five times per week. It is imperative for good healing that between treatment sessions, the patient carries out some home exercises to further optimize the tensile strength of the new scar formation. Such exercises are also clearly described by McKenzie.

I. Effects

Deep transverse friction (DF) has three main effects:

- Traumatic hyperemia, which helps evacuate pain-triggering metabolites.

- Movement of the affected structure, which prevents or destroys adhesions and helps optimize the quality of the scar tissue.

- Stimulation of mechanoreceptors, which produces a quantity of afferent impulses that stimulate a temporary analgesia. This also helps the patient to perform movement exercise.

II. Indications

The indications are muscular, tendinous, and ligamentous lesions.

III. Contraindications

The contraindications include:

- Calcification,

- Rheumatoid tendinous lesions,

- Local sepsis, and

- Skin diseases.

IV. Technique

A. Exact Localization

It is imperative that DF is given at the site of the lesion; after all, that is where we need to influence the scar formation.

B. No Movement Between Finger and Skin

We need to friction the structure and not the overlying skin. Do not glide over the skin; doing so might damage the skin, making DF impossible for the subsequent session(s).

If the patient used a creamy body lotion, then cleanse the skin with alcohol or use a thin layer of cottonwool between the finger and skin.

C. Transverse

DF is given transverse to the fiber direction.

D. Sufficient Amplitude

We must be sure to make a large movement and move over, up, and again over the structure in order to have good contact. Therefore, it is necessary to take a reserve of skin; we first move the skin superficially in the opposite direction and then apply pressure and perform the active phase of the DF.

E. Sufficient Depth

How deep must the deep friction be? It must be sufficient to reach the structure, so it depends on the structure's location.

F. Starting Position

Make sure the friction massage is comfortable for you as well for the patient. Position the patient in such a way that you can easily reach the structure to which you want to apply friction. Adopting a comfortable position will also save energy.

Make the lesion accessible to the finger. Tendons with a tendon sheath are generally frictioned in a stretched position, just like ligaments (so as to make better contact).

Muscle bellies are always frictioned in a shortened position (making it easier to move the fibers in relation to each other).

G. Grips

Various grips are used according to the nature and the position of the lesion.

H. Economy of Effort

Concentrate on performing an arm movement instead of a small finger movement, since this is much more comfortable for the patient and for the therapist.

The movement should have two phases: an active phase with more pressure (movement of the structure) and a relaxation phase without pressure.

Always try to keep your finger joints slightly flexed (if you friction too much with your interphalangeal joints in hyperextension, you might provoke a traumatic arthritis in those joints).

V. Duration, Frequency

For most lesions, three times per week is sufficient frequency. The duration is usually 15 minutes per session, but the first session should be limited to 10 minutes. In some chronic lesions, the duration of treatment will reach 20 minutes. If more than one area has to be treated (e.g., Achilles tendinitis), it will be 10 minutes per localization.

There are two exceptions that call for use of a different strategy: the medial collateral ligament of the knee and the lateral ankle ligaments. Here, the deep friction is given in a progressive way. The details will be discussed in the appropriate sections.

If the structure is too tender on palpation, the interval between the sessions is prolonged; the duration and the intensity of the deep friction do not change.

The treatment can be ended when the patient is symptom-free and the functional examination has become negative; any remaining local tenderness on palpation can be ignored.

Exception—Quadriceps and hamstrings muscle bellies. To avoid recurrence, the treatment has to be continued for another week after full clinical recovery.

VI. Normal Execution

When describing the techniques in detail, the phrase "the deep friction is executed in the normal way" will often be mentioned. What we mean by that is: one or more fingers are placed onto the lesion, reinforced by one or more fingers. A reserve of skin is taken in the opposite direction; pressure is applied, and the active phase of the deep friction is then a movement in the direction of the therapist. In most cases, this is a large arm movement rather than a small finger movement, with all the finger joints slightly flexed. The relaxation phase then follows in the opposite direction.

Remark—Sometimes all the fingers are used next to each other for DF (e.g., when treating muscle belly lesions in large muscles). This is necessary to prevent the formation of adhesions. When the deep friction is given tenoperiosteally, there should always be contact with both tendon and bone.

I. Capsular Stretching

This technique is used in the first stage of an arthritis (the first 2 weeks and the last few months). It consists of reaching the end of range and stretching for about 45 seconds, then relaxing and stretching again.

A treatment consists of capsular stretching for 10 mintues, followed by mobilization for another 10 minutes, three times a week; home exercises in which the end of range is regularly reached must also be incorporated.

The amount of stretching is appropriate if the patient reports 2-3 hours of discomfort after treatment. Thus, we inquire about the patient's reaction at the next session: no post-treatment soreness means stretching was insufficient; too much post-treatment soreness means stretching was too forceful.

Photo 1

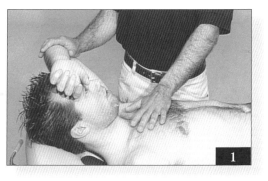

II. Distraction

In the third stage of an arthritis, the distraction technique is used purely for pain inhibition, and not for mobilization (too painful). Under slight traction, barely visible vibrations are applied for about 20 minutes. The patient's shoulder is kept in a comfortable position to ensure that the therapist can work without causing the slightest pain. To prevent adaptation of the nervous cells, minute changes are constantly built in (rhythm, starting position).

Frequency—Four to five times a week, without exercises or mobilization.

In the second stage of an arthritis, the distraction technique is adapted to the obtained result:

- Stage II+: It becomes more of a mobilization.

- Stage II–: The joint is now mobilized at the end of the possible range in every direction.

Photo 2

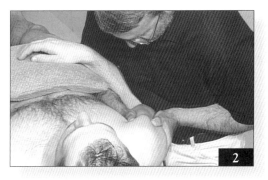

III. Deep Friction, Acromioclavicular Joint

The therapist palpates cephally in the deltoid area until reaching the lateral edge of the acromion. The joint line lies 1 to 1.5 centimeters more medially.

The deep friction is performed in the normal way with the ipsilateral index finger, reinforced by the middle finger. A large amplitude is required.

3

Shoulder: Techniques

Photo 3

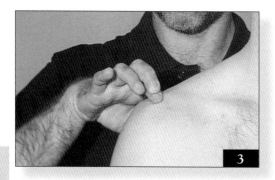

structure. Don't be confused by this fact; poor vascularization of the tenoperiosteal area may be the cause of this discrepancy in symptoms.

Photo 4

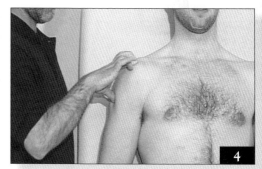

IV. Deep Friction, Supraspinatus, Tenoperiosteal Junction

The patient sits with his arm behind his back (medial rotation makes the insertion of the tendon, now lying in front of the acromion, accessible to the finger). We can palpate the spine of the scapula in a lateral direction; as soon as we lose contact with the bone, we come back onto the bone and palpate, this time in an anterior direction. We know for sure that we are on the acromion. The tendon, with its insertion on the greater tuberosity, is located just beyond the anterior edge of the acromion.

The deep friction is performed in the normal way, with the index finger of the ipsilateral hand, reinforced by the middle finger. The thumb should be placed quite far down the arm. To exert a downward pressure on the greater tuberosity, the index fingernail should remain horizontal. (If the thumb were to be placed posteriorly, with the nail of the index finger pointing anteriorly, pressure would be exerted on the front of the acromion and the lesion would be missed. This is a frequent error.)

There may be minor tenderness on palpation, with more tenderness lateral and medial to the

V. Deep Friction, Supraspinatus, Musculotendinous Junction

For this technique, the patient's arm rests in about 90° of abduction. The therapist stands at the opposite side and uses the middle finger of the ipsilateral hand, reinforced by the index finger. The therapist palpates the space between the spine of the scapula and the clavicle toward the lateral direction, looking for tenderness. The palpation is a pronation/supination movement with a flexed middle finger.

This deep friction is an exception to the general rule because it has two active phases instead of an active and a relaxation phase. We use the middle finger to obtain equal range in both directions. Be sure to perform a large movement and avoid extending the distal interphalangeal joint (otherwise you will be unable to maintain good contact and could also damage your own interphalangeal joint).

Photo 5

Photos 6 through 8

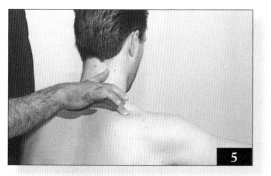

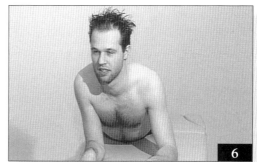

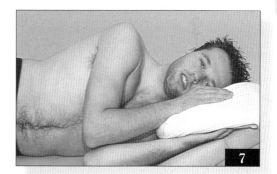

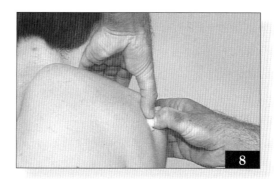

Shoulder: Techniques

VI. Deep Friction, Infraspinatus

The patient is treated in the sphinx position (prone on elbows): 90° of elbow flexion with the shoulder in slight lateral rotation and adduction. Although this is the best position, it is not always the most comfortable (e.g., elderly patients or some back patients). For that reason, there is an alternative in side-lying where the same components as in the sphinx position can be built in.

Technique—To find the precise location, the palpation consists of a supination movement with the thumb flexed. In this way, when palpating under the spine of the scapula in a lateral direction, the difference between muscle belly (soft), tendinous body (cable), insertion (cable and bone), and beyond the insertion (bone without cable) can clearly be felt.

The deep friction itself begins by taking a reserve of skin in a pronation direction, then applying pressure and performing the active phase of the movement, which is a supination. Since the skin in this area is very vulnerable, a thin layer of cottonwool is used between the patient's skin and the frictioning thumb.

It is best to perform this technique with both hands, whereby one thumb reinforces the other. Make sure the frictioning thumb remains flexed, or you will loose good contact.

VII. Deep Friction, Subscapularis

Palpation—For a right subscapularis, we palpate under the clavicle with the left thumb in a lateral direction until reaching the coracoid process. We then move caudally and laterally again until we feel the lesser tuberosity (*check:* lateral to this bone, we find the bicipital groove).

With the thumb well flexed and pointing toward the nipple at a 45° angle, we make a large movement forward (taking the skin along) and then move back to the lesser tuberosity. The purpose is to keep a deltoid border behind our finger so that we can reach the structure in a more optimal and direct way. While performing this backward movement, we can feel one or two tendons slip under our thumb (short head of biceps and coracobrachialis), and if we keep our thumb flexed, we will not lose the anterior edge of the deltoid muscle. We then bring our thumb back in a longitudinal direction for the deep friction.

The technique will consist of a large rolling movement of the arm cephally, keeping the thumb as flat as possible for the patient's comfort. However, a slight degree of flexion is permanently needed to keep the edge of the deltoid behind our thumb during the entire friction. Therefore, we cannot release the pressure completely on the way back, as in a normal deep friction.

Photo 9

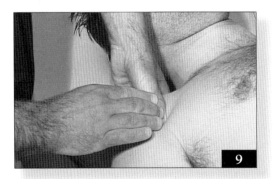

VIII. Deep Friction, Long Head of Biceps in the Bicipital Groove

Palpation—See the technique for the subscapular tendon.

With the patient's arm in lateral rotation, the contralateral thumb is placed into the groove longitudinally and pressure is exerted sideways. The active phase of the deep friction is a medial rotation with the other arm while the thumb exerts pressure.

Remark—The groove can easily be felt, but the tendon is not always felt (likely depends on the height of the bony edges of the groove).

Photo 10

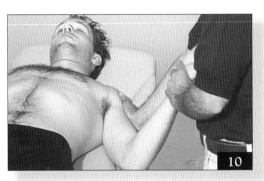

I. Manipulation for Loose Body

Assistants—Ideally, two assistants take care of fixating the patient. One immobilizes the patient's distal arm (preferably with the palm of one hand on that of the other hand); the second assistant steadies the patient's shoulder (toward the table) and his lower ribs (toward himself). If necessary, the first assistant's foot also provides a fulcrum for the therapist's foot.

If no assistant is available, it may be possible to fixate the patient using a belt.

Photos 11 through 14

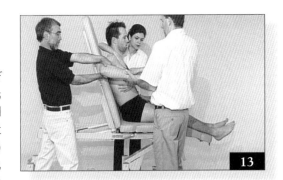

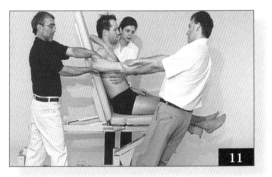

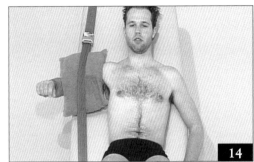

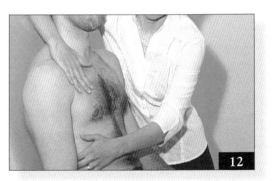

Grips—Two different grips are used, one for a pronation and one for a supination maneuver.

- Pronation: For a right elbow, the right hand grasps the radius in pronation; the other hand applies strong pressure on the first hand to prevent gliding over the patient's skin.

- Supination: The right hand now grasps the radius in supination; the other hand acts as before.

4

Elbow: Techniques

4

Photos 15 through 18

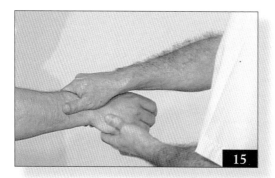

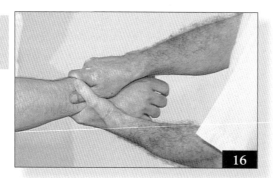

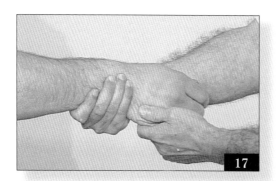

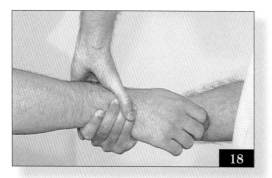

Execution—For a right elbow, the therapist stands on his left foot and, with both arms extended, applies traction using his body weight. He pivots from about 100° to 170° (the extension limitation should not be exceeded) and, during this movement, performs three full rotations toward pronation or toward supination. The last rotation is combined with a right side bending of the trunk (to get an extra traction impulse).

It is important to perform full rotations and to return to the neutral position each time; less than full rotations have no effect. There should always be a visual control to prevent exceeding the limit of range.

In practice, one manipulation is performed, followed immediately by a control. We assess the range of extension. Then a second manipulation is performed, again with a control. In this way, some 10-12 manipulations are done in one session, if necessary (mostly pronations and some supinations; we choose supination when pronation ceases to help). A complete result is expected in about two sessions. The treatment ends as soon as extension is free again and the normal hard end-feel is felt again.

II. Deep Friction, Muscle Belly of Biceps

With the muscle in a relaxed position, the precise site of the lesion is found on palpation. The deep friction consists of a pinching technique; the fingers are applied anteriorly to the muscle and a reserve of skin is taken in a posterior direction. Then pressure is applied (the pinch is closed, as it were) and the active phase is a movement straight forward, during which we can feel the fibers of the biceps slide under our fingers. Avoid making a circular movement and flexing the interphalangeal joints too much.

Photo 19

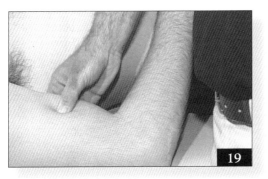

IV. Deep Friction, Triceps

The starting position for this technique is 90° of flexion and supination. The deep friction is executed in the normal way with one to three fingers, depending on the size of the lesion, and with the thumb acting as a fulcrum anteriorly.

Photo 21

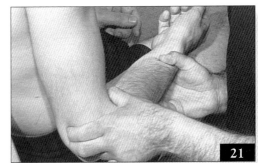

III. Deep Friction, Insertion of Biceps

We palpate the joint line between the humerus and radius. Two centimeters more distally, the flexed thumb is applied quite medially, with the patient's arm in supination. The thumb is set in sharply and deeply.

The active phase of the deep friction consists of bringing the patient's arm into pronation while exerting pressure with the thumb. At around three-quarters of pronation, the biceps insertion slips under our thumb. The pressure is released on the way back. Some discomfort during this friction is normal.

Photo 20

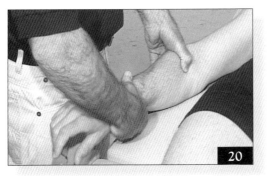

V. Deep Friction, Supinator

Here, the starting position is three-quarters of extension and pronation. We find the precise spot by palpating in the zone between the radius and ulna. For a right elbow, the flexed left thumb is used between the radius and ulna. (Avoid placing the thumb cranial to the radius, in the extensor muscles.) A reserve of skin is taken in an oblique cranial direction. The deep friction is an active movement in an oblique downward direction. It is a smooth arm movement rather than a pure thumb movement. Notice that not much space is available.

Remark—Make sure you have space to perform an arm movement during the frictioning.

Photo 22

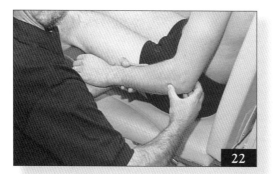

the lateral epicondyle; we put our thumb a little bit higher until we reach the sharp edge just above the lateral epicondyle. We flex the thumb to 90° so that the thumbnail now faces forward. A reserve of skin is taken upward, and pressure is applied on the anterior aspect of the humerus. The active phase of the deep friction is an arm movement downward with pressure in a posterior direction, followed, as always, by a phase of relaxation.

Photo 24

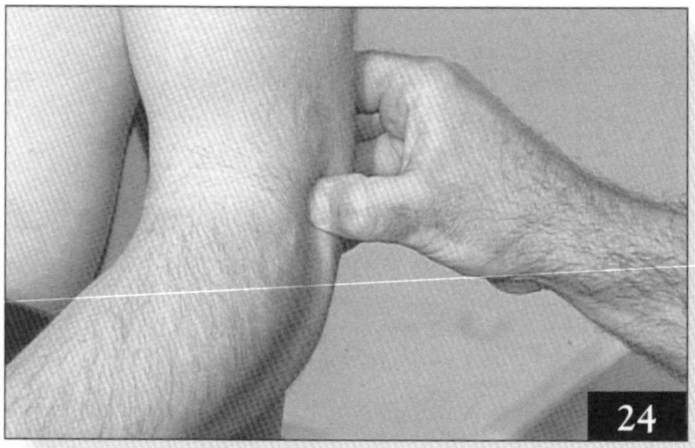

VI. Deep Friction, Pronator Teres

During palpation, we ask the patient for a slight contraction toward pronation to make sure that we find the correct structure. The deep friction is done in the normal way.

Photo 23

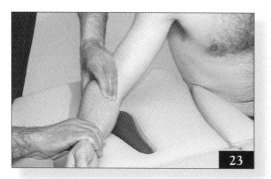

VII. Deep Friction, Extensor Carpi Radialis Longus (Type 1)

The starting position is 90° of elbow flexion and supination. We palpate the lateral aspect of

VIII. Deep Friction, Extensor Carpi Radialis Brevis, Body of Tendon (Type 3)

The starting position is three-quarters of extension and pronation. First, we look for the precise location: the tendon level with the joint line or with the radial head. The thumb is placed as flat as possible on the lesion; a reserve of skin is taken in a medial direction, and pressure is applied. The active phase of the deep friction is a movement in a lateral direction.

Photo 25

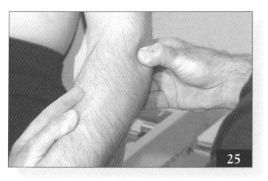

IX. Palpation, Extensor Carpi Radialis Brevis, Muscle Belly (Type 4)

The starting position is 90° of flexion and supination. Level with the neck of the radius, we use a pinching grip with all fingers; the muscle belly is lifted upward, as it were. This automatically results in a visible wrist extension.

Photo 26

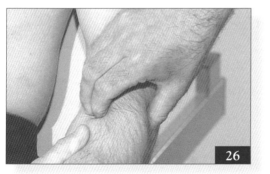

X. Deep Friction, Extensor Carpi Radialis Brevis, Tenoperiosteal Junction (Type 2)

The starting position is 90° of flexion and supination. The therapist's thumb is flexed to 90°, with the tip of the thumb lateral to the lateral epicondyle. The deep friction must be applied at the front of the epicondyle, so the therapist then brings his thumb onto the anterior aspect of the bone. The correct spot is reached when only a very small range of movement is possible (a translation movement in a medial direction) and when the movement stops with a harder end-feel. The other fingers act as a fulcrum at the medial side of the elbow. The active phase of the deep friction is a translation movement at the front of the lateral epicondyle, with pressure applied in a medial/downward direction.

To avoid losing contact with the lesion, the patient should not abduct his arm, nor should the therapist's thumb be in too high or too flat a position.

Using a layer of cottonwool between the frictioning finger and the skin will help prevent damage to the skin (short fingernails are an advantage).

Photo 27

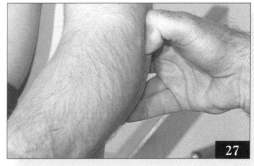

XI. Mill's Manipulation

Always start by checking the range of extension; 180° is a minimum (185°-190° is acceptable). Three elements must be built into the procedure: maximal wrist flexion (the patient's arm in medial rotation and the therapist's thumb between the patient's thumb and index finger), maximal elbow extension, and finally, a step sideways behind the patient's back. The latter element is necessary for maintaining the maximal wrist flexion.

The therapist stands at the posterior aspect of the patient, with the proximal foot at the height of the patient's shoulder.

The maneuver is performed in four steps: first, medial rotation at the shoulder, followed by wrist flexion, elbow extension, and last, a small step sideways. These elements have to be coordinated, with the manipulation itself becoming a combination of the last three elements. Notice that the manipulation is performed with very high velocity, very small amplitude, and without any strength at all. The crack heard on manipulation has no therapeutic value.

Photo 28

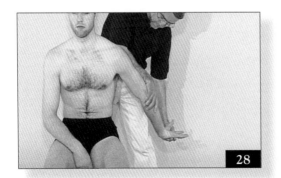

XII. Deep Friction, Golfer's Elbow

With the patient's elbow in full extension, we locate the medial epicondyle and proceed to the front of it. Deep friction is executed in the normal way.

Remark—

- At the tenoperiosteal junction, the deep friction is a straight-line movement and the feel is rather hard;

- At the musculotendinous junction, the deep friction is a more ample rounded movement and the feel is softer.

Photo 29

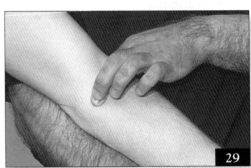

I. Carpal Subluxation, First Manipulation

For this procedure, an assistant stabilizes the distal part of the patient's arm and, with his foot, can provide a fulcrum to the therapist.

Grip—For a right wrist, the therapist's right thumb is placed distally on the radius and ulna; the left thumb lies on the carpus. Both thumbs are parallel. The therapist's left fifth finger maintains the patient's wrist in a middle position.

Execution—The therapist faces away from the patient in order to build in some traction at the wrist. He stands on one leg, using part of his body weight in an oblique direction, and performs a few antero-posterior gliding movements.

After each attempt, the range of passive extension is assessed.

Photos 30 and 31

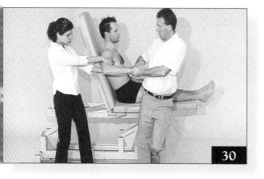

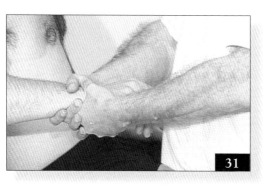

Remark—The patient also can be fixed using a strap.

Photo 32

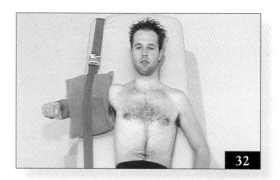

II. Carpal Subluxation, Second Manipulation

5

The assistant's role is the same as for the first manipulation.

Grip—For a right wrist, the left thumb is placed transversally on the metacarpal bones. The therapist's right hand squeezes the wrist.

Execution—Same as for the first technique. The manipulation is a quick, strong squeeze.

Photos 33 and 34

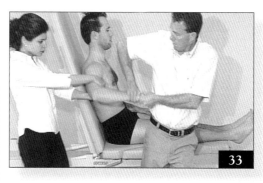

Wrist and Hand: Techniques

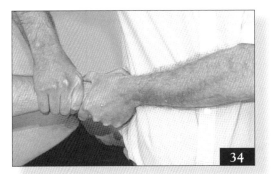

The following alternative eliminates the need for an assistant and does not require fixation of the upper arm. Stand with your back toward the patient and make precise contact on the desired carpal bone (e.g., capitate and lunate); build in traction and perform an antero-posterior gliding movement.

Photo 35

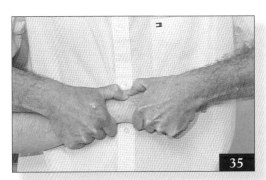

III. Carpal Subluxation, Third Manipulation

When no assistant is available, the first maneuver can be done as follows. The patient's hand is positioned beyond the edge of the table so that he can immobilize his lower forearm himself by grasping the lower edge of the table. The therapist holds one bone (e.g., the capitate) between both thumbs and both index fingers, steps slightly backward for the traction component, and performs a very localized antero-posterior glide.

Photo 36

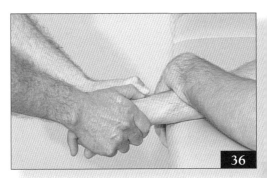

IV. Carpal Subluxation, Fourth Manipulation

Another way of performing the first maneuver, maintaining the same grip and performing the same manipulation, is for the therapist to build in traction by pushing his knee comfortably against the patient's arm.

This manipulation can also be performed more specifically with a precise contact on one or more bones.

Photo 37

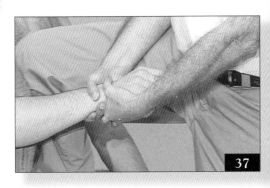

V. Deep Friction, Dorsal Ligament in the Proximal or Distal Row

The patient's wrist is held in flexion. The therapist sits at the patient's ulnar side, close to the treatment table; the patient's arm is positioned slightly beyond the edge of the table. For a right wrist, the deep friction (lateral-medial) is performed in the normal way with the right index finger, reinforced by the middle finger.

Photo 38

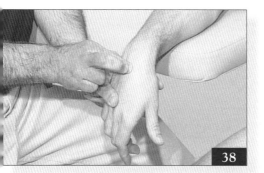

VI. Deep Friction, Dorsal Ligament in the Middle Row

The wrist is held in flexion; the therapist faces the patient. The deep friction (cephal-caudal) is performed in the normal way using the tip of the thumb.

Photo 39

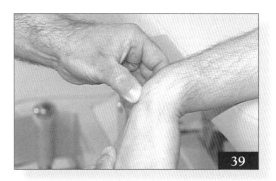

VII. Deep Friction, Extensor Carpi Radialis Longus or Brevis

The therapist sits at the patient's ulnar side, close to the treatment table. The patient's arm is slightly beyond the edge of the table; the wrist is held in flexion. Deep friction is executed in the normal way using the index finger, reinforced by the middle finger.

The longus inserts radially on the base of the second metacarpal bone; the brevis inserts radially on the base of the third metacarpal bone.

Photo 40

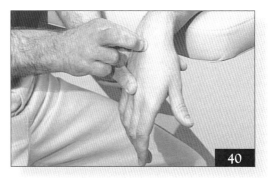

5

Wrist and Hand: Techniques

VIII. Deep Friction, Extensor Carpi Ulnaris

The wrist is held in radial deviation. The deep friction is executed in the normal way using the index finger, reinforced by the middle finger.

Photo 41

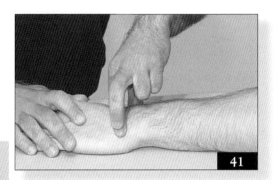

X. Deep Friction, Flexor Carpi Ulnaris

The wrist is held in extension; the deep friction is executed in the normal way using the thumb.

Photo 43

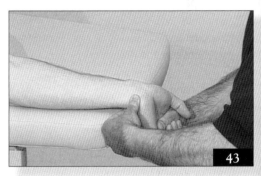

IX. Deep Friction, Flexor Carpi Radialis

The wrist is held in extension; the deep friction is executed in the normal way using the thumb.

Photo 42

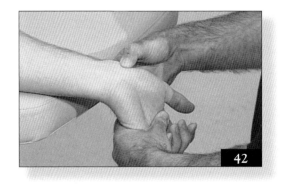

XI. Deep Friction, Flexor Digitorum Profundus

The wrist and the fingers are held in extension. The deep friction is executed in the normal way using four fingers, with the thumb acting as a fulcrum.

Photo 44

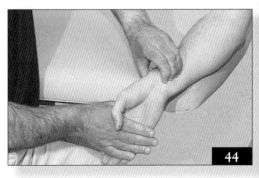

XII. Deep Friction, Anterior Part of the CMC I Joint

Palpation of the joint can be done as follows. During passive abduction and adduction or flexion and extension movements, we palpate the first metacarpal bone in a proximal direction; first, we feel only bone; then we reach the joint line, and consequently we feel movement. This is the joint line between the trapezium and the first metacarpal.

For a left hand (palm facing upward), the right thumb is positioned at the front of the joint and the thenar muscle is pushed aside. The capsule is slightly stretched by an extension-backward movement of the patient's thumb. The active phase of the deep friction is a supination movement of the forearm. The patient's hand should be positioned beyond the edge the table so that there is enough space for the therapist's arm to perform the movement.

Photo 45

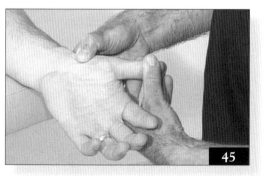

XIII. Deep Friction, Lateral Part of the CMC I Joint

Changing from the anterior to the lateral part of the joint is accomplished as follows. The patient's hand is brought into a vertical position; the therapist changes thumbs (to allow the previously used thumb to relax for 5 minutes), moves laterally, and stretches the capsule by bending the patient's thumb. The deep friction is executed in the normal way.

Photo 46

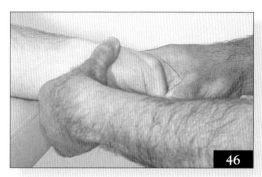

5

Wrist and Hand: Techniques

XIV. Deep Friction, Tenosynovitis, Tunnels 1 and 3

The patient's wrist and thumb are flexed. The therapist's thumb is placed longitudinally onto the lesion. A large reserve of skin is taken toward pronation, after which the deep friction consists of a supination movement with the ipsilateral hand.

Photo 47

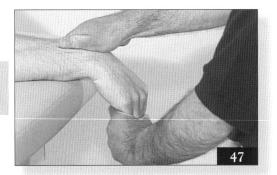

XV. Deep Friction, Interosseous Muscle Belly

The patient's hand lies flat on the table with the fingers slightly spread. This deep friction is an exception to the two-phase rule (active phase followed by a relaxation phase). The deep friction, which is performed using a slightly bent middle finger, is a pronation-supination movement in which the pressure is not released (i.e., both movements are active phases).

Photo 48

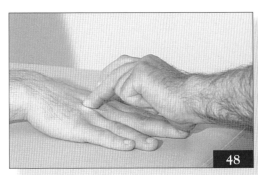

XVI. Deep Friction, Interosseous Tendon

To reach this somewhat palmarly situated tendon, we have to create some room for our thumb. We use our middle finger to push one knuckle in an upward direction and our thumb to push the other knuckle downward. The deep friction consists of a supination movement using the tip of the thumb.

Photo 49

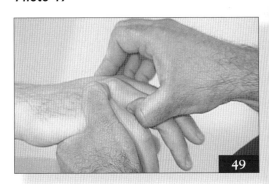

I. Capsular Stretching in Flexion

In this maneuver, the therapist uses one hand to immobilize the patient's other leg, and builds in hip flexion using his body weight through the other hand. The capsule is stretched for 45-60 seconds, either intermittently or sustained.

Photo 50

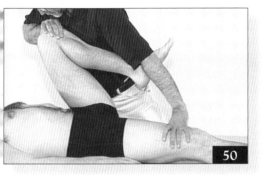

Photo 51

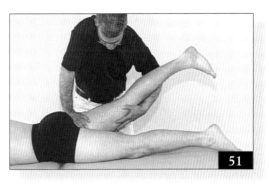

III. Capsular Stretching in Extension, Second Technique

In this variant, the patient's thigh rests on the therapist's thigh. This enables the therapist to use more of his body weight (building in a side flexion).

II. Capsular Stretching in Extension, First Technique

One hand is positioned on the upper femur and the other hand just above the knee. The capsule is stretched by using the therapist's body weight.

Photo 52

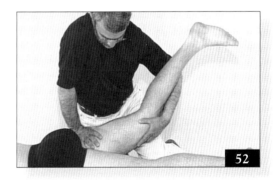

Remark—Excessive knee flexion should be avoided in order to avoid too much stress on the quadriceps.

6

Hip: Techniques

IV. Capsular Stretching in Medial Rotation

The therapist stabilizes the patient's pelvis with one hand and with his other hand grasps the leg on the same side, just above the ankle. Using this lever, the capsule is stretched in medial rotation. The therapist should be mindful of the relaxation of the adductor muscles.

Photos 54 through 56

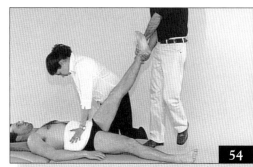

Photo 53

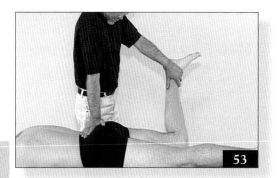

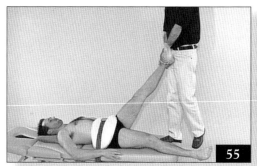

6

Hip: Techniques

V. Loose Body, First Manipulation

The patient's pelvis is stabilized by an assistant or by a strap. The therapist stands on the end of the table, grasps the patient's ankle, and holds the limb in approximately an 80° straight-leg raise. Using a grip that prevents excessive movement in the foot, the therapist uses his body weight to apply traction in this 80° SLR direction; he maintains this traction while gradually stepping backward off the table. In the meantime, during the "flight phase," he performs three full rotations (medial or lateral).

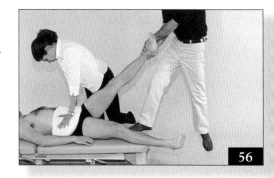

- *Grip for medial rotation:* The therapist faces medially and uses his distal hand to grasp the lateral malleolus; his proximal hand supports and stabilizes the grip.

- *Grip for lateral rotation:* The therapist faces laterally and uses his distal hand to grasp the medial malleolus; his proximal hand supports and stabilizes the grip.

Photos 57 and 58

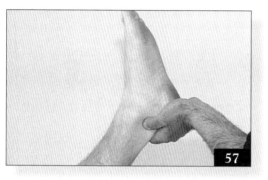

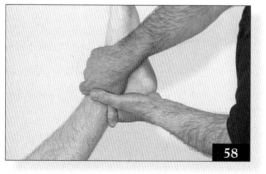

VI. Loose Body, Second Manipulation, Medial Rotation

Photo 59

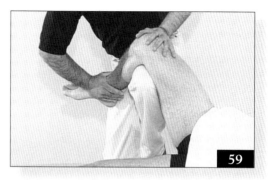

Execution: See VII.

VII. Loose Body, Second Manipulation, Lateral Rotation

The patient's pelvis is stabilized by an assistant or by a strap. For a right hip, the maneuver is as follows: The therapist puts his left foot on the table and, by means of an abduction movement, positions his thigh under the patient's knee (comfortably; i.e., not under the calf). With the patient's knee now bent, an assistant stabilizes the patient's pelvis, and the therapist half plantarflexes his foot. He leans sideways to increase the traction component, maintaining the knee flexion while reaching the end of medial or lateral rotation. The manipulation consists of a high-velocity, low-amplitude jerk toward rotation combined with the second half of plantarflexion at the therapist's foot.

- *Grip for medial rotation:* The therapist has one hand on the outer part of the knee and one hand medially above the foot.

- *Grip for lateral rotation:* The therapist has one hand on the inner part of the knee and one hand laterally above the foot.

Photo 60

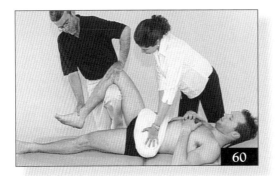

Remark—A technical problem may arise when the therapist is either much taller or much shorter than the patient. In the former case, he sets his leg obliquely instead of vertically; in the latter case, he needs to have a platform under his foot.

VIII. Deep Friction, Adductor Longus, Musculotendinous Junction

The starting position for this maneuver is with the patient's leg in slight abduction and lateral rotation. The deep friction is a pinching technique with the thumb and fingers, with the heel of the hand acting as a fulcrum. A large reserve of skin is taken in a lateral direction, then pressure is applied; the active phase of the deep friction consists of a horizontal movement in a medial direction.

Photo 61

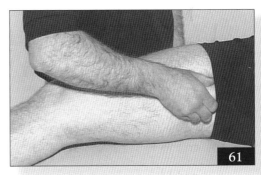

IX. Deep Friction, Adductor Longus, Tenoperiosteal Junction

The starting position for this maneuver is with the patient's leg in slight abduction and lateral rotation. For a right adductor longus, we palpate in the cranial direction with the left middle finger until we feel the inferior edge of the pubic bone; the finger is then turned 45° medially and now feels bone and tendon at the same time. The frictioning finger is reinforced by the other middle finger. The deep friction is executed in the normal way.

Photo 62

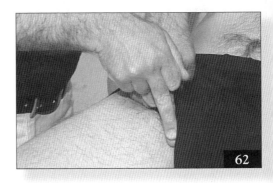

X. Deep Friction, Psoas Muscle Belly

The patient adopts the half-lying position. The lesion is located below the inguinal ligament and medial to the sartorius muscle. For a right psoas muscle, we use the right index and middle fingers, reinforced by the left middle and ring fingers. Make sure that during the deep friction you maintain a deep contact.

Photos 63 and 64

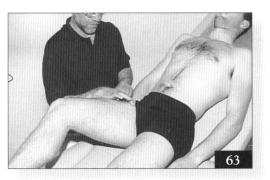

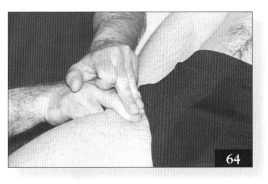

Remark—For the patient's comfort, it is essential to keep the fingers horizontal and to increase the pressure gradually.

XI. Deep Friction, Rectus Femoris Tendon

The patient sits in 90° of hip flexion. We locate the tendon just lateral to the sartorius muscle. For a right rectus femoris, the flexed fingers of the left hand, reinforced by the fingers of the other hand, grasp the tendon. The deep friction is executed in the normal way with an active phase toward the therapist.

Photo 65

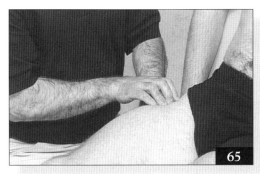

XII. Deep Friction, Iliotibial Band

The patient lies on his side with a cushion between his knees. The therapist takes a reserve of skin toward himself, then places his thumb onto the lesion and reinforces it with the heel of his other hand; both arms are extended. The deep friction is performed in the normal way, in which the active phase is a forward movement of the entire trunk. The patient's pelvis is stabilized by the therapist's thigh and fingers.

6

Hip: Techniques

6

Hip: Techniques

Photos 66 through 68

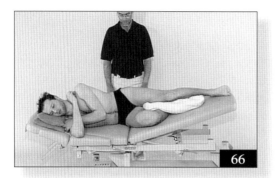

66

Photo 69

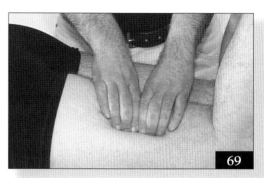

69

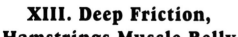

67

XIV. Deep Friction, Origin of Hamstrings

The patient lies on his side with the hips and knees in 90° of flexion. The deep friction is executed in the normal way with two or three fingers; the fingers feel the ischium and the tendons at the same time.

Photo 70

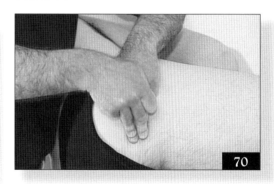

70

68

XIII. Deep Friction, Hamstrings Muscle Belly

The muscle is in a fully relaxed position (patient lying prone, knees in 90° of flexion). The deep friction is executed in the usual way with all fingers, covering a large area so as to limit the risk of adhesion formation.

Remark—It is easier to work in close contact with the patient on a higher treatment table.

I. Meniscus Manipulation

This maneuver is a short thrust toward extension with both hands, combined with valgus and medial rotation components.

Execution—One hand grasps the knee (thumb at the back) and the other hand is positioned at the heel. The therapist repeatedly extends the knee by stepping sideways while avoiding the painful end of range; then valgus is added (by stepping backward). We build in three to four full medial rotations without losing the valgus component. The final thrust is a swift coordination of all these elements.

Photo 71

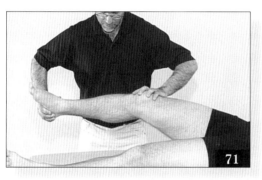

II. Loose Body: Basic Manipulation

The patient lies prone.

Grip—For a right knee, the left index finger is placed on the tibia, the palm of the hand facing upward. The right hand is placed along the Achilles tendon and brings the foot into dorsiflexion (to stabilize the ankle joint).

Execution—The therapist puts his left foot on the table and brings the patient's foot onto his thigh. The assistant then pushes the patient's thigh down onto the table, thus applying traction. Keeping the patient's foot raised as long as possible, the therapist steps sideways, using his body weight. At the same time, he performs three full

rotations. (He chooses either medial or lateral rotation (it doesn't matter which); depending on the result, one or the other is repeated.)

Remark—If the patient's leg is too long compared to therapist's leg, the therapist can position a phone book under his foot.

It is also possible to employ this technique without an assistant, by using a strap.

Photos 72 through 74

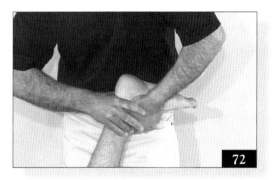

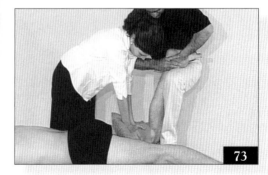

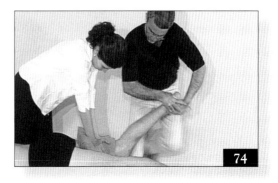

7

Knee: Techniques

III. Loose Body: Flexion Manipulation

The therapist uses his wrist as a fulcrum at the back of the patient's knee and performs a high-velocity, low-amplitude flexion manipulation.

Photo 75

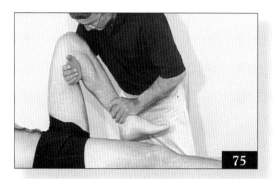

Photos 76 and 77

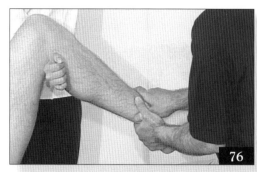

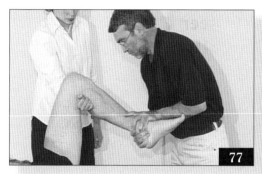

IV. Loose Body: Flexion-Rotation Manipulation

An assistant's wrist is positioned behind the patient's knee. The manipulation consists of three rotations (medial or lateral) during a flexion movement. The flexion component is executed by the therapist's trunk, the rotations by his hands.

- *Grip for lateral rotation at the left knee:* The therapist sits medial to the patient's foot. His right hand grasps the medial malleolus in pronation; his left hand supports and immobilizes the patient's leg.

- *Grip for medial rotation at the left knee:* The therapist stands lateral to the patient's foot. His left hand grasps the lateral malleolus in pronation; his right hand supports and immobilizes the patient's leg.

V. Loose Body: Extension-Varus Manipulation

Grip for the right knee—The therapist's left hand is positioned proximal to the knee (thumb anterior and fingers medial). The right hand is placed just proximal to the foot (thumb anterior and fingers lateral). As a maximum varus strain is applied, we ask the patient to actively straighten the knee while we maintain the pressure toward varus. At the end of range, both hands perform a short thrust toward extension.

7

Knee: Techniques

Photo 78

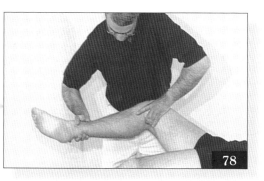

VI. Deep Friction, Medial Collateral Ligament

The friction is applied in as much extension and flexion as possible. The knee is supported by a cushion. For a left knee, we use the left middle or index finger; we locate the joint line and palpate in a posterior direction until the ligament (a large flat structure) is found beyond the midline. The deep friction is executed in the normal way.

For the deep friction in flexion, we first find the lesion in extension and, keeping our finger on it, bend the knee. Again, the deep friction is executed in the normal way. Notice that the direction in which the ligament now lies has changed, and so has the direction of our friction.

Photos 79 and 80

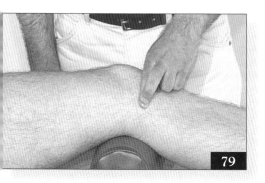

VII. MCL: Manipulation Toward Flexion

This maneuver consists of a few preliminary flexion movements followed by a thrust toward flexion.

Photo 81

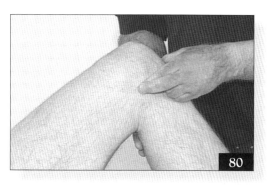

VIII. MCL: Manipulation Toward Medial Rotation

The patient's knee is supported by the therapist's shoulder. The heel is grasped with both hands; full medial rotation is repeated a few times, followed by a thrust.

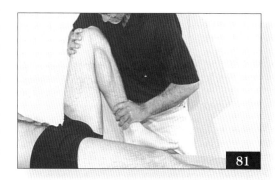

7

Knee: Techniques

Photo 82

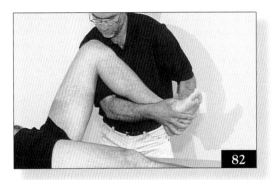

IX. MCL: Manipulation Toward Lateral Rotation

The starting position is three-quarters of flexion. With our forearm, we bring the foot into dorsiflexion, then use the medial border of the foot as a lever to reach full lateral rotation. After a few preliminary lateral rotations, a thrust follows.

Photo 83

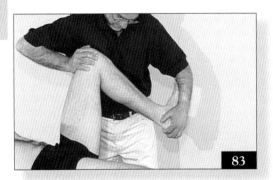

X. MCL: Manipulation Toward Extension

One hand is placed just proximal to the knee, the other just proximal to the foot. Both thumbs face anteriorly. The hand next to the knee performs a preliminary flexion-extension movement, which is followed by a high-velocity, small-amplitude thrust with both hands toward extension.

Photo 84

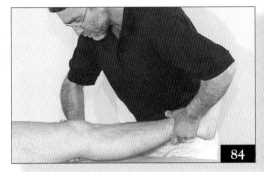

XI. Deep Friction, Lateral Collateral Ligament

With the patient's knee extended, we palpate the joint line in a posterior direction. We feel, successively, bone, then a thin flat structure (iliotibial tract), bone again, and then a tendon-like structure, the LCL. Even more laterally, the biceps tendon can be found.

The deep friction is executed in the normal way.

Photo 85

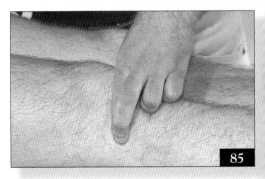

XII. Deep Friction, Medial Coronary Ligament

The starting position is with the patient's knee in 90° of flexion and lateral rotation. For the left knee, we place the left index finger onto the tibial plateau. The fingernail faces upward; in this way, pressure can be applied in a downward direction. The thumb should be placed far down so as to maintain this pressure. The deep friction is executed in the usual way.

For a lateral coronary ligament, the knee is positioned in medial rotation.

Photos 86 and 87

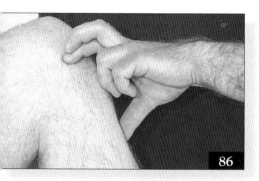

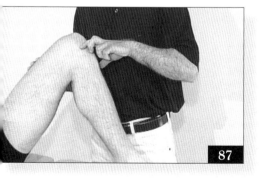

XIII. Deep Friction, Quadriceps Muscle Belly

The muscle is in a shortened position (i.e., the patient is in a seated position without a cushion under the knee). Large contact is made with both hands; the deep friction is executed in the normal way with all fingers. The active phase of the DF is reinforced by a backward movement of the trunk; the relaxation phase is a forward movement.

Photo 88

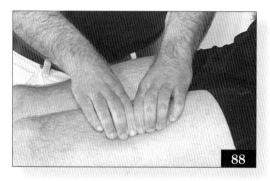

XIV. Deep Friction (Tenoperiosteally), Supra- and Infrapatellar Tendinitis

Suprapatellar—The distal half of the patella is pushed in a posterior direction so as to make the proximal part tilt forward, which makes it easier to reach the lesion. The deep friction is executed in the normal way with the ring finger, reinforced by the middle finger, using the thumb more distally as a fulcrum. The pressure is applied toward the toes.

Since the lesion lies tenoperiosteally, there is contact with the contractile structure and the bone at the same time.

7

Knee: Techniques

Infrapatellar—In this case, the upper half of the patella is pushed posteriorly. The deep friction is the same as for a suprapatellar lesion.

Photos 89 through 91

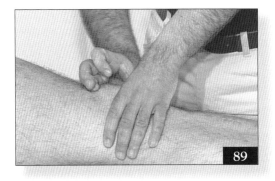

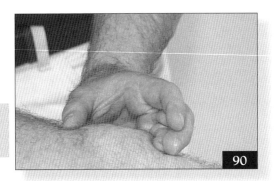

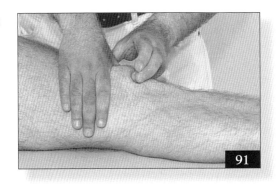

XV. Deep Friction, Medial Quadriceps Expansion

For a left knee, the right thumb pushes the patella in a medial direction. The left hand is in supination; the ring finger, reinforced by the middle finger, exerts an anterior pressure on the back of the patella.

The deep friction is executed in the normal way (i.e., a reserve of skin is pushed in a cranial direction, then pressure is applied; the active phase is a caudal movement with pressure in an anterior direction). It is an arm rather than a finger movement. The forearm remains parallel to the patient's leg. For practical reasons, the deep friction is done in a caudal direction.

Photo 92

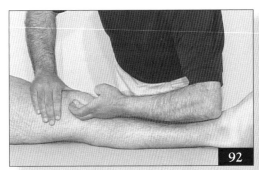

XVI. Deep Friction, Iliotibial Band

The structure is found halfway between the infrapatellar tendon and the LCL. The lesion lies at one of three possible sites: at the joint line or either slightly above or below it. The deep friction is performed in the normal way across the fibers

Photo 93

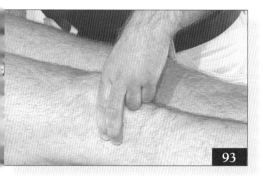

XVII. Deep Friction, Biceps Femoris Tendon

The patient lies prone with his foot beyond the edge of the table. He actively holds his foot up for a moment to enable us to find the tendon more easily. The deep friction is executed in the normal way with one, two, or three fingers, according to the size of the lesion.

Photo 94

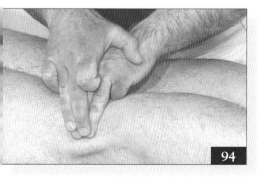

XVIII. Deep Friction, Pes Anserinus

We palpate the soft structures from distal to proximal until we find the bony edge of the tibia;

then we move I centimeter distally again. The fingers are applied in a 45° medial-downward direction. The deep friction is executed in the normal way with four fingertips, reinforced by the other hand.

Photo 95

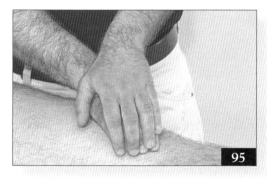

XIX. Deep Friction, Popliteus Muscle Belly

The patient lies prone with his knee slightly bent. We first palpate the head of the fibula, then I.5 centimeters cephally up the joint line, and another I.5 centimeters cephally lies the insertion on the lateral femoral condyle. From there, we imagine a 45° line caudally, and the muscle belly lies fanwise around this line.

We look for the most tender spot, pull the reserve of skin toward us, and apply the flattened thumb to the lesion, reinforced by the heel of the hand. The therapist's arms are kept straight. The deep friction consists of an active phase medially upward, followed by a relaxation phase. It is more a trunk movement than an arm movement. So as to work comfortably, the pressure is only gradually increased.

7

Knee: Techniques

Photos 96 and 97

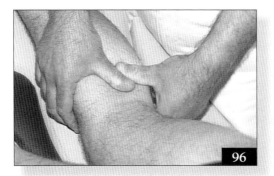

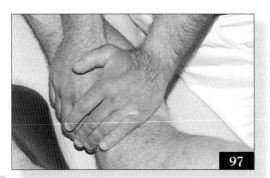

friction is performed by either the left or the right thumb (therapist's choosing). The tip of the thumb is placed vertically into the sulcus; the active phase of the deep friction is a transverse movement toward the left or the right.

The sulcus can always be felt, but it may not be possible to feel the tendon.

Photos 98 and 99

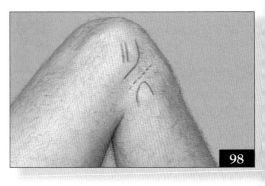

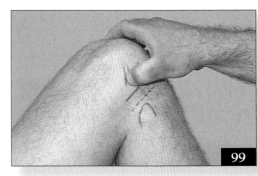

XX. Deep Friction, Popliteus Insertion

The starting position is with the patient's knee in 90° of flexion. About 1 centimeter from the edge of the femoral condyle, we find a vertical sulcus containing the popliteal tendon. The deep

7

Knee: Techniques

8

I. Deep Friction, Gastroc-nemius Muscle Belly

The starting position is with the patient's foot in plantarflexion and the knee slightly flexed. The deep friction is carried out in the normal way, using all fingers, regardless of the size of the lesion. This technique significantly minimizes the risk of adhesions. Be sure to take enough reserve of skin so that the range of movement can be large enough. The DF movement can be guided by a body movement.

Photo 100

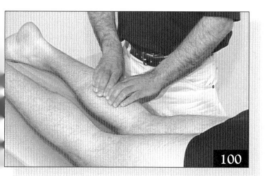

II. Deep Friction, Achilles Tendon, Medial/Lateral Aspect

The therapist can either stand or sit. His thigh immobilizes the patient's foot in dorsiflexion in order to bring some tension into the tendon. The DF is a pinching technique with the thumb and index finger, reinforced by the middle finger. A large reserve of skin is taken in an anterior direction, then pressure is applied; the active phase of the DF is a straight movement backward. For the patient's comfort it is important that the therapist's DIP joints are not flexed too much. To avoid damage to the skin, a thin layer of cotton wool should be used between the fingers and the skin.

This maneuver is best performed with both hands simultaneously. After pushing the skin forwards, the therapist's arms are almost extended.

Photo 101

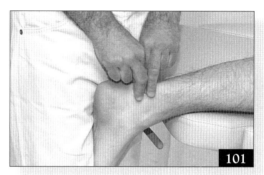

III. Deep Friction, Achilles Tendon, Anterior Aspect, Medial

In plantarflexion, the tendon is pushed medially by the therapist's thumb to create the necessary space for frictioning. The contact with the thumb is not sharp, but flat. The DF is performed with the ring finger, reinforced by the middle finger. First, a reserve of skin is taken in pronation, then pressure is applied; the active phase of the DF is a supination movement.

It is very important that the therapist's forearm remains parallel to the patient's leg. Thus, the couch should be in a rather high position to enhance the therapist's comfort.

8

Photo 102

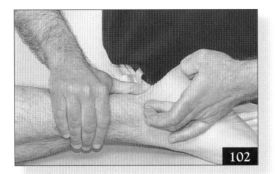

IV. Deep Friction, Achilles Tendon, Insertion

Again, the starting position is with the patient's foot in plantarflexion. The DF is executed in the normal way with both index fingers. The fingers and thumbs form a circle, and pressure is applied toward the toes. The finger feels tendon and bone at the same time.

Photo 103

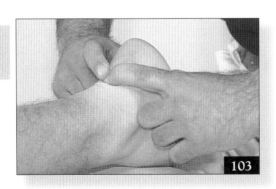

V. Deep Friction, Peronei, Above the Malleolus

The therapist stands next to the patient. The tendons are stretched by some plantarflexion and adduction. The DF is executed in the normal way

with one or more fingers (depending on the size of the lesion).

Photo 104

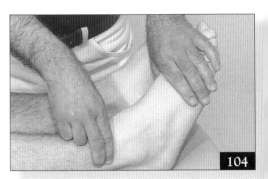

VI. Deep Friction, Peronei, Below the Malleolus

The starting position is the same as for the previous maneuver. The DF is executed in the normal way with the index finger, reinforced by the middle finger.

Photo 105

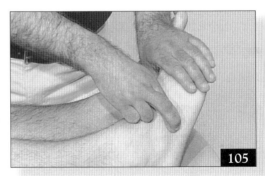

VII. Deep Friction, Peronei, Behind the Malleolus

Again, the tendons are in a stretched position. The therapist, however, now stands in front of the patient. This part of the tendon is treated with a supination technique with the ring finger, reinforced by the middle finger. All finger joints are slightly flexed. A reserve of skin is taken in pronation; the active phase of the DF is a supination movement.

Photo 106

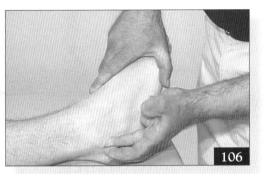

VIII. Deep Friction, Tibialis Posterior, Below the Malleolus

The tendon is stretched by bringing the foot into dorsiflexion. The DF is executed in the normal way with one or two fingers, depending on the size of the lesion.

Photo 107

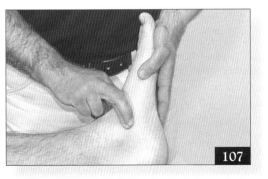

IX. Deep Friction, Tibialis Posterior, Above the Malleolus

The therapist's thigh keeps the patient's foot in dorsiflexion. The entire ring finger is placed on the lesion and a reserve of skin is taken in pronation; pressure is applied, and the active phase of the DF is a supination movement. Reinforcing the ring finger with the fingers of the other hand makes the active phase even more effective and certainly more practical.

Photo 108

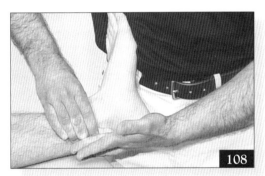

X. Deep Friction, Anterior Talofibular Ligament, Fibular Insertion

The ligament is stretched by a plantarflexion-adduction-supination movement. We palpate the ligament along the fibular edge. The DF is executed in the normal way with the index finger, reinforced by the middle finger, and the thumb acting as a fulcrum. The thumb is positioned such that the DF is given in a 45° direction to the foot. The index finger feels bone (fibula) and ligament at the same time.

8

8

Photo 109

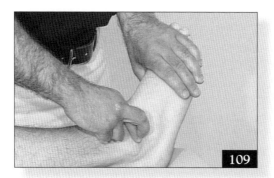

XI. Deep Friction, Anterior Talofibular Ligament, Talar Insertion

The starting position is the same as for the fibular insertion. By changing the position of the thumb, the DF is now given in a 90° direction to the foot (instead of the 45° of the previous maneuver). The index finger feels the talus and ligament at the same time.

Photo 110

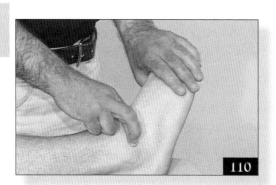

XII. Deep Friction, Calcaneofibular Ligament

The homolateral hand keeps the heel in varus. The DF is executed in the normal way with the ring finger, reinforced by the middle finger, and the thumb acting as a fulcrum. The thumb is placed anteriorly on the patient's leg such that the direction of the DF is toward the patient's heterolateral shoulder. The finger has contact with both ligament and bone.

Photo 111

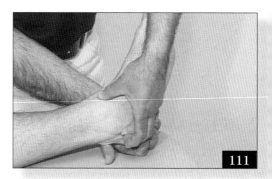

XIII. Deep Friction, Calcaneocuboid Ligament

The foot is kept in some midtarsal adduction. *Palpation*—The therapist stands medially to the patient's foot and places his heterolateral thumb first on the head of the fifth metatarsal bone, then next to it (proximal); the joint line between the cuboid and calcaneus now lies just proximal to the therapist's thumb. The index finger palpates along the joint line from the sole to the dorsum of the foot; first, a peroneal tendon is felt, then bone, and eventually a flat, soft structure, which is the calcaneocuboid ligament.

The DF is executed in the normal way with the index finger, reinforced by the middle finger, and the thumb acting as a fulcrum.

Photo 112

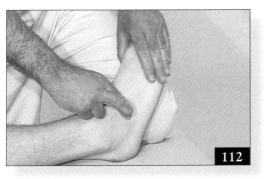

112

XIV. Manipulation, Lateral Ligaments

For rupturing ligamentous adhesions, several components need to be built in to end range: varus at the talocalcanean joint, plantarflexion at the ankle joint, adduction, and supination. When these components are built in, the manipulation is executed by a small adduction at the shoulder joint. The rupturing of the adhesions can usually be heard.

During the next few days, the patient's regained mobility needs to be maintained by general mobilization.

Photo 113

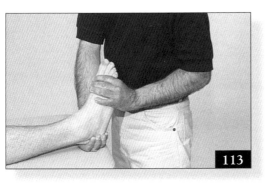

113

XV. Loose Body Manipulation, Ankle Joint

An assistant stabilizes the patient by holding his arms.

Grip—For a right foot, the therapist's left hand holds the calcaneus; the right hand grasps the forefoot. A reserve of skin is taken until the little finger makes contact with the talus. The therapist's feet are braced against the couch and his toes point to the right.

Execution—With the left hand on the patient's heel, the left foot braced against the leg of the couch, the right hand on the patient's forefoot, and the right foot against the couch, the therapist bends at the knees and straightens his arms, then performs several deep knee flexions (i.e., three consecutive movements of sitting down and raising slightly up again).

This maneuver can and may only be performed when the patient's muscles are completely relaxed.

Photo 114

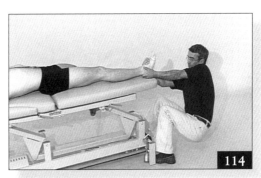

114

XVI. Loose Body Manipulation, Talocalcanean Joint

The starting position for this maneuver is with the patient lying prone with his foot over the edge of the couch. He performs an active dorsi-flexion and pulls himself up until the dorsum of the foot touches the edge of the couch. He then moves upward another inch or so.

Grip—Both thenars are placed medially and laterally on the calcaneus. The fingers are crossed at the dorsum of the foot. The therapist stands close to the couch, with his legs slightly spread and his elbows pointing outward. Using his body weight, he builds in traction and then performs several energetic varus-valgus movements.

Remark—Be sure you perform a varus-valgus and not a rotation movement.

Photo 115

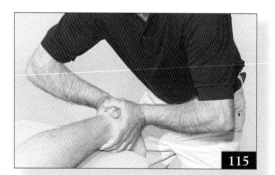

8

XVII. Mobilization for Metatarsus Inversus

For a right foot, the grip is as follows: The heel of the therapist's left hand is placed on the plantar aspect at the outer forefoot, the heel of the right hand dorsally on the inner forefoot. The ankle joint is stabilized by leaning well forward, and the forefoot is mobilized toward lateral rotation.

Photo 116

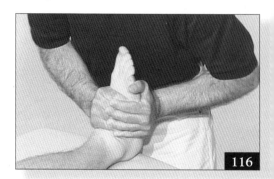

XVIII. Cuboid Rotation Manipulation

This maneuver is a manipulation of the cuboid bone in a dorsal/lateral direction with the patient lying prone or standing.

Photo 117

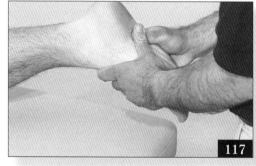

I. Indications

"Any disc protrusion in the absence of contraindications."

The only goal of theraputic manipulation is to bring about a reduction of the internal derangement. This means that both the lesion and the patient should be amenable to manipulation.

Any strategy must be based on signs and symptoms and response to movement. After reducing the internal derangement, we must ensure that it stays reduced and that the patient can recover full function. Prophylaxis and self-treatment procedures will also play important roles.

Preferably, the protrusion should be annular, not too large (no motor or sensory deficit), and not located too far lateral. The patient should not be overly nervous and should want to get well.

To relax the patient, we should thoroughly educate him on the nature of the problem and the procedure to be performed. Involving the patient makes it easier for him to understand the purpose of the treatment and some self-treatment procedures.

Generally speaking, reduction by manipulation is possible in two-thirds of all cases of backache and in one-third of all cases of sciatica. Thus, in about half of the cases, performing manipulation could be beneficial. To determine which cases are suited for manipulation and which are not, we must interpret the findings of the history and the clinical examination.

A. Indications from the History

1. How did the symptoms start?

Was there sudden onset (during a movement), or did the symptoms applear gradually over the course of some hours or days? A pain appearing suddenly suggests an annular (harder) protrusion, making it more suitable for manipulation.

2. Age

Due to changes in the water content of the disc, manipulation becomes even more efficient as age advances.

3. Primary posterolateral protrusion

This is almost always a softer protrusion (it is seen mostly in young patients) and is therefore more suitable for traction than for manipulation.

4. Nuclear self-reducing disc protrusion

Reduction is not the problem, as the protrusion reduces spontaneously on decompression. This is a case for stabilization and self-treatment.

5. The mushroom phenomenon

This is also a compression phenomenon and is unsuitable for manipulation.

B. Indications from the Examination

1. Acute lumbago

   a. Good indication, except if highly irritable

If we are barely able to examine the patient (too much pain, almost no movement is possible), we think of an epidural local anesthesia first, after which the patient should remain in bed and try to perform movements in decompression. One or two days later, he should be much better and can be reexamined and manipulated if necessary.

   b. Nuclear acute lumbago: "nuclear manipulation"

In the nuclear variant of acute lumbago, traction is only indicated in theory. In practice, the pain is much too acute; the patient feels more comfortable during the traction, but when the traction force is released, he develops severe pain and is unable to get up from the table for an hour or more.

The best we can do is to manipulate in a nuclear manner; when, the end of range is reached, instead of using the manipulative thrust,

Lumbar Manipulation

9

we keep the patient in this position, as relaxed as possible, for about 10 seconds (i.e., incorporating a certain stretch that has a traction component). We repeat this technique eight or nine times, possibly with some slight rhythmical stretching maneuvers, so as to obtain a gradual reduction.

c. With/without deviation

Deviation automatically means that the protrusion is larger (i.e., that more sessions will be required to achieve a lasting reduction).

2. Backache

The following elements are very favorable:

- A sudden onset,
- A minor partial articular pattern,
- Favorable articular signs (see Part I), and
- The presence of a painful arc.

Remark—This type of clinical image will most likely respond very quickly with manipulation.

A deviation will make obtaining a reduction a little more difficult but still possible.

3. Root pain

- It is better if the patient is not too young.
- Other favorable elements include:
  - If some backache remains,
  - If the root pain is recent,
  - Minor or no deviation,
  - Favorable articular signs (see Part I),
  - Only slight limitation of SLR, and
  - No neurological deficit.

4. Elderly patient

- Manipulation is more indicated than continuous traction.

- We should, however, adapt our techniques to the patient's age:
  - Perform only three to four maneuvers in a session.
  - Allow a longer interval between sessions (twice a week?).
  - Avoid techniques with a lever because of potential fractures.

5. Mixed protrusion

- One or two sessions of manipulation, followed by further treatment with traction.

II. Contraindications

Manipulation is contraindicated in the following cases:

1. If the lesion is not a disc protrusion/internal derangement.

2. If there is no protrusion at the moment.

3. If there is excessive tension in the posterior longitudinal ligament:

- S4 symptoms or signs,
- Bilateral sciatica, or
- Spinal claudication (see Part I). Here, the history is typical: unilateral or bilateral sciatica after walking for some time.

4. The use of anticoagulants is an absolute contraindication (due to the risk of an intraspinal hematoma). In the history taking, we always inquire about the use of medication. If there is the slightest doubt about the effects of a drug, the therapist should inquire. Prolonged steroid treatment, possibly resulting in osteoporosis, is also a contraindication for certain manipulation techniques.

5. If there is an aortic graft.

6. During pregnancy:

   • No manipulation in the last month.

   • No extension techniques (in prone lying) after four months.

7. For the "neurotic" patient. Such patients always respond unfavorably to manipulative/active treatment.

Manipulation is unlikely to succeed in the following cases:

1. If the pain is too severe.

2. If the protrusion is too large:

   • Neurological deficit (note that this is not always an indication for surgery).

   • Sciatica with extreme deviation laterally or in flexion.

3. If the protrusion is too soft (nuclear).

4. If the root pain has existed for more than 6 months in a patient under 60 years of age. The protrusion has become irreducible (over half of the period of the spontaneous cure), and manipulation will probably fail (see Part I).

5. If there are compression phenomena: mushroom phenomenon, nuclear self-reducing disc protrusion.

6. If a protrusion at the same level after laminectomy seems to have a stronger nuclear character.

7. If there are unfavorable articular signs (see Part I).

8. If there is a primary posterolateral protrusion.

III. Choice of Techniques

A. General Hints

• Techniques with a lever should be avoided in elderly or osteoporotic patients (this is also true for young patients who have had large, long-standing doses of steroid drugs).

• Rotation techniques usually work very well for an L4 protrusion. For an L5 disc, extension techniques occasionally can be better. The reason might be that anatomically there is less rotation between L5 and S1 than between L4 and L5.

• Extension techniques should not be used for an acute lumbago (the patient is fixed in flexion, so manipulation toward extension would be very painful).

• The "stretch" technique (see later discussion) is always the first technique to be performed in a treatment session (mainly because of its longitudinal traction effect).

• Several maneuvers are performed in a manipulation session. A normal "dose" for a young adult is about seven to nine maneuvers in a session. For an elderly patient, three to four maneuvers will suffice, and the interval between the sessions is longer. A young patient can come back the next day if necessary, whereas an elderly patient requires 3 or 4 days between sessions.

We never know in advance how many maneuvers will be necessary. It depends entirely on the patient's reaction.

A. Basic Rules

There are a number of basic rules:

• Each maneuver is first done at half the normal intensity.

- There is a retest control after each maneuver; we retest the test(s) that were positive in the examination in order to assess the evolution. (Which tests? SLR if positive, articular lumbar movements in standing if SLR is negative.)

- A maneuver that helps the patient is repeated.

- A maneuver that does not help is abandoned.

- We should only increase the intensity of a maneuver if the less intense version has proved beneficial.

- If a maneuver ceases to afford further benefit, another maneuver is chosen, again starting at half the intensity.

The therapist does not know at the start of a treatment session which techniques he will use and how many times; it depends entirely on the evolution of the patient's symptoms and signs, which are the most important factor for treatment success and therapist guidance.

D. Interpreting Improvement

What can be interpreted as an improvement?

- Less pain.

- Increased range of movement (although the pain may be unaltered). In this case, it might be interesting to perform the lumbar movements in standing before a mirror so that the patient can see the improvement for himself.

- Fewer movements are painful.

- A "shortening" of the pain (i.e., the lesion centralizes). In this case, the patient may experience this subjectively as a worsening because he feels pain in a location where

he didn't feel pain before (example: leg pain that changes into gluteal and then back pain). We should inform the patient about the positive interpretation of this centralization.

- The appearance of a painful arc.

Remark—A maneuver that makes the patient worse or that causes pain in the limb should not be repeated.

The above-described indications and contraindications are very detailed and to the point; they are meant to increase the safety and efficiency of our procedures. We are able to relieve the patient of his pain quickly, and then we must make sure to incorporate self-treatment elements to optimize the long-term result.

IV. Techniques

A. Rotation Manipulation: Stretch

Starting position—The treatment table should be as low as possible (if possible, a maximum height of 45 centimeters). For a unilateral pain, the patient lies on the painless side. For a central pain, he can lie on either side, or a choice is made according to which SLR is worse (if known). The lower limb is extended and the upper limb is flexed, with the foot behind the back of the other knee.

Grip—The therapist has one hand behind the greater trochanter with the fingers pointing caudally and the other hand at the front of the shoulder with the fingers pointing cephally. His feet are spread apart. Contact is made with the skin in order to avoid gliding.

Three components must be built in. The first is shoulder and pelvic rotation, with both rotations being equal. Then the therapist adds a longitudinal taking up of the slack, rising onto his tiptoes and using his body weight precisely above the patient's trunk with his arms extended. This taking up of the slack is followed almost immediately by the manipulative thrust; while maintaining the distraction, part of the therapist's body weight is used as a pelvic swing in a longitudinal direction (the direction of the flexed upper limb of the patient).

In the nuclear variant of the stretch, no thrust is used; the patient remains in the distracted position for up to 15 seconds, and after two to three repetitions, the effect is assessed. The maneuver can then be repeated.

Remark—Eperience shows that not every patient responds optimally to the stretch maneuver with the painful side upward. Occasionally, it is better to open the painless instead of the painful side. The reason is unclear; we think that the biomechanical pressure forces within the disc, as well as whether the annular wall is intact or not, could play an important part in this.

Photos 118 and 119

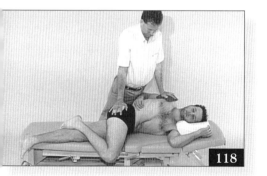

118

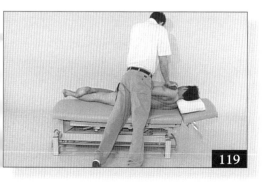

119

B. Rotation Manipulation with Lever: Leg-Over

Starting position—The correct supine position of the patient should be estimated; if the patient lies too far toward the opposite side, the leg will catch the treatment table during the manipulation, blocking the manipulative movement. If the patient lies too close to the therapist, he will fall off the table. Thus, we look for a midposition. The therapist stands at the pain-free side.

Execution—Assuming that the right side is the painful one, the therapist grasps the patient's right knee with both hands, flexes the hip to about 90°, and under traction (to make it more comfortable for the patient) brings the patient's knee to well below the edge of the table (the patient's left hand lies on his abdomen). The patient will feel as though he is going to fall off the table and will try to keep himself from doing so. This is not necessary; the therapist only applies a slight counterpressure against the patient's shoulder. The patient's thigh should not be braced against the edge of the table; if necessary, he should be moved a bit more toward the therapist (positioning of the patient is critical). Thus, the therapist brings the knee far down, turns his hand outward, and stands with both legs apart, facing the patient's feet.

Taking up the slack is performed as follows: the therapist brings his right foot against his left one (he ceases to straddle) and applies his body weight to the patient's right shoulder to reach the end of range. He makes sure that the knee remains down so as not to lose the slack. The manipulative thrust is a sudden push downward with the hand on the knee.

For an upper lumbar protrusion, more hip flexion is needed.

Lumbar Manipulation

9

Photos 120 and 121

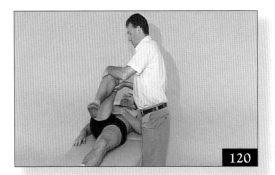

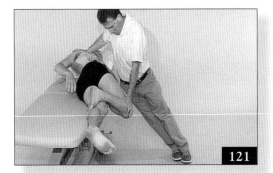

C. Rotation–Side Flexion Manipulation: Dallison

This is a specific technique that can be used when the patient has pain and a lateral deviation. The maneuver is actually a combination of a leg-over and a side flexion. The logic behind it is as follows. A patient with a deviation to the left spontaneously opens the right hand side at the lumbar level because he feels better in this position. So the therapist does the same and accentuates it; he also opens the right side by means of a left side flexion. It is immaterial whether the pain is left or right; what matters is which side the patient opens spontaneously. We are guided by the patient's position.

Starting position—The patient should be in the correct supine lying position (see leg-over). If the therapist wants to build in a side flexion to the left, he stands at the left side of the table and crosses the patient's left knee over the right one; his left hand grasps the back of the patient's right knee, and his right hand is placed at the outer aspect of the left knee. Both hips are flexed, and a side flexion to the left is built in using a "swing" movement and maintained.

The rest of the maneuver is the same as for the leg-over: bringing the knee far down without losing too much hip flexion, exerting body weight on the patient's shoulder, and manipulation with the hand on the knee.

Photos 122 and 123

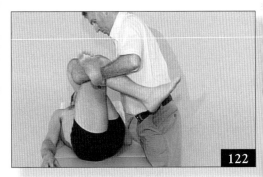

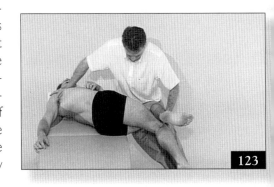

D. Rotation Manipulation: Reverse Stretch

Starting position—The table should be as low as possible (preferably lower than 45 centimeters). The patient lies on the pain-free side, with the lower arm behind his back. The upper arm is relaxed in front of him, with the hand hanging off the edge of the table. The upper limb is brought backward and hooked on the edge of the table.

Execution—The therapist stands in a cranial direction, and again the slack is taken up in rotation; both rotations should be equal. The therapist uses one hand, fingers directed upward, against the anterior superior iliac spine to obtain pelvic rotation and maintains it by extending his elbow. With the other hand against the spine of the scapula, he builds in the other rotation.

The second element is the distraction; the therapist faces the patient's head, rises onto his tiptoes, and uses his body weight above the patient in a longitudinal direction. The manipulative thrust is a downward jerk toward distraction using the body weight.

Remark—This maneuver is unsuitable for obese or very stiff patients who do not have much pelvic rotation. A platform can be used if the therapist has difficulty bringing his body weight above the patient (tall patient, short therapist).

Photos 124 and 125

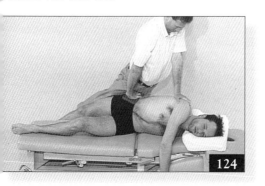

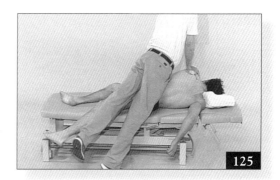

E. Extension Manipulation: Central Pressure

Starting position—The table is at knee height; the patient lies prone.

Grip—First, the middle of the fifth metacarpal bone is applied vertically between two spinous processes, reinforced by the other hand, and then the lower hand is brought in an almost horizontal position for the patient's comfort.

Execution—The therapist leans against the table with his feet spread apart and his arms extended. Part of his body weight takes up the slack, and the manipulative thrust toward extension, again using the body weight, follows. Make sure that the arms remain extended at all times.

Remark—If during the taking up of the slack, the patient feels a pain in the buttock or the limb, the maneuver should be abandoned. It is important not to lose the slack just before the manipulative thrust.

Lumbar Manipulation

9

Photos 126 and 127

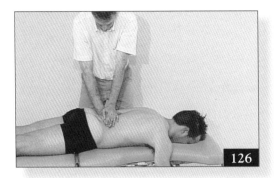

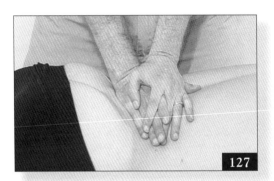

F. Extension Manipulation: Unilateral Pressure

Starting position—The same as for the central pressure manipulation. The patient should not lie in the middle of the table, but should be positioned as close as possible to the therapist. The therapist should be positioned on the patient's right side for a left unilateral pressure.

With the pisiform bone positioned on a transverse process, a slight reserve of skin is taken toward the midline. Then the paraspinal muscles are pushed away laterally and the hand is pulled backward to make a bony contact as close to the midline as possible, thus avoiding the risk of fracture of a transverse process (because of its thin

shape). Using his other hand to reinforce the grip, the therapist then leans forward, with his shoulders well beyond the midline; to maintain his balance, he slides down with his legs against the edge of the table.

Part of the therapist's body weight takes up the slack; the manipulative thrust is performed with straight arms in a medial and caudal direction.

Remark—The patient should be positioned very close to the therapist.

Photo 128

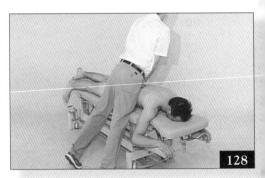

G. Mobilization: Stretch in Prone Lying

Starting position—With the patient lying prone, the painful side is opened by means of a trunk side flexion.

Execution—Taking a reserve of skin, the therapist places his hands (arms crossed) against the lower ribs and the iliac crest. With both legs extended well backward, he lies on the patient. The maneuver (a mobilization rather than a manipulation) is a rhythmic posteroanterior pressure (four to five times) of the thorax with elbows bent 90°, thus distracting the painful side

Photo 129

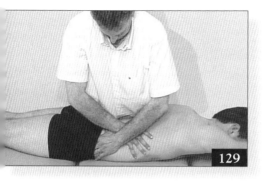

H. Deviation Reduction Technique, Rotation

Starting position—The patient lies on the convex side (e.g., on the left side for a deviation to the right). The lower limb is extended, the upper limb is flexed with the foot behind the other knee, and the knee hangs beyond the edge of the table.

Execution—The therapist stands in front of the patient, immobilizing his knee, and leans with his body weight onto the patient's shoulder in a combined rotation and distraction direction. A very strong traction is felt; it is maintained for up to a minute, then released and repeated again.

Remark—The patient needs to lie as much as possible on the edge of the table.

Photo 130

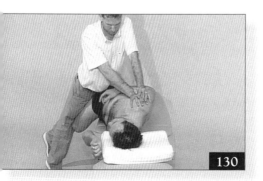

I. Deviation Reduction Technique, Side Flexion

In a left deviation, side flexion toward the right is limited. This is the direction that will be mobilized.

Starting position—The patient lies supine; the therapist stands at his right side and crosses the right knee over the other one.

Execution—The therapist move his right hand under the patient's right knee and over his left knee and grasps the back of the left knee. The hips are brought into flexion. The therapist's left hand is at the outer aspect of the patient's right knee. In this way, by swinging with both hands, rhythmic side flexion movements toward the right are performed; occasionally, the end of range is maintained for a while.

Photo 131

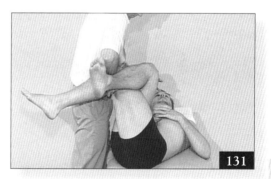

J. Deviation Reduction Technique, Extension

Starting position—The therapist stands at the side of the deviation and with both hands grasps the patient's other pelvis.

Execution—The therapist pushes with his trunk and pulls with the arms in order to first neutralize and then correct and overcorrect the deviation. A movement toward extension follows; it is maintained for a few seconds and performed three times in succession. For maintaining balance, the therapist should push the patient slightly forward during the extension and should accompany this movement by side flexing his trunk. He should also position his knee in front of the patient's knee to prevent the patient from doing too much knee flexion during the extension.

Remark—If the patient is too tall in relation to the therapist, the maneuver can be done with the patient sitting at the distal edge of the table, with the legs fixed with a strap.

Photos 132 and 133

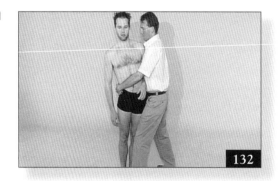

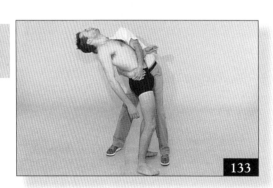

V. Manipulative Strategy

Depending on the patient's response to our manipulative strategy, there are multiple strategies (tracks) that can be followed.

As stated earlier, a manipulation always starts with a stretch at low intensity with the painful side up.

A. First Track

A **stretch** is performed, followed by checking the SLR (or any other positive lumbar movement in standing if the SLR is negative). If the patient's condition is improved, the stretch is repeated, again with a control afterward. As long as the maneuver is beneficial, it is repeated with increasing intensity. We never know in advance how many times to repeat the maneuver. The number of repetitions depends entirely on the patient's symptoms and signs.

Eventually a point is reached where the patient is already much better but the last maneuver has ceased to afford further benefit. How is this to be assessed? The stretch technique is no longer beneficial; we should now continue with a technique that goes in the same direction as the previous rotation: *the* **leg-over**. It is performed at low intensity first, then repeated a few times. If after six to eight maneuvers, the patient is much improved, the therapist can decide to end the treatment session and to continue the next day or the day after.

Remark—At the next session, the therapist does not continue with the last technique used at the end of the previous session. Instead, he must reassess because the protrusion may have migrated, and thus the session starts with the stretch again, followed by interpretation of the result. This is actually an **"open-ended" strategy**.

It is interesting to note that often only the stretch and the leg-over are needed to obtain full recovery (specifically, in small internal derangements with favorable articular signs).

There is a variant of this first track for a patient with pain as well as deviation: the use of the **Dallison** technique will play a role. We take into consideration that five or six sessions will be required instead of three or four to obtain reduction. In each session, we might use the stretch two to three times, the leg-over two to three times, and finally the Dallison technique one to two times.

Another variant is the case where the patient with pain and deviation no longer has pain after a few sessions but the deviation remains relatively unchanged. The three anti-deviation techniques (deviation reduction) are then indicated. The mechanism of the painless deviation is still unclear, as is the true biomechanical effect of the **anti-deviation techniques**. Those techniques are based on a hypothetical empirical experience.

This first track is apparently a very positive track, but adaptations are sometimes necessary.

B. Second Track

If a low-intensity stretch was unsuccessful, there is a tendency to make two mistakes: to perform a more forceful stretch or to try a leg-over (which is an intensified version of the stretch). However, it makes much more sense to try the other rotational direction and to proceed with a low-intensity **reverse stretch**. If this maneuver helps, it is repeated a few times until it ceases to be beneficial.

This second track is needed less frequently than the first one.

C. Third Track

As always, we start with the stretch, which may or may not be beneficial. If it helps, we repeat it several times; if not, we do it only once. In any case, a point will be reached where we will have to choose a second technique: the **central pressure**. Why?

- Because the patient is elderly or osteoporotic, has an osteoarthrotic hip, or has had a total hip replacement; in all these cases, the thigh cannot be used as a lever, so the leg-over is contraindicated.

- Because the patient has an L5 disc protrusion, which might respond better to an extension than to a rotation technique.

- Another reason may be that the patient has good extension and very painful flexion in standing. Hence, taking up the slack in extension is likely to be comfortable, whereas for a leg-over it could be rather uncomfortable. Thus, we choose the more comfortable technique.

On this third track, the techniques are used in the following order: **central pressure, unilateral pressure on the pain-free side first, then on the painful side, and the stretch in prone lying** to end the session.

It is possible that taking up the slack for the central pressure will produce pain in the limb. If it does so, this technique should be disregarded and the unilateral pressure used.

Lumbar Manipulation

9

I. Effects

Traction is a way of increasing and accelerating the moderate decompression obtained with recumbency. Several authors confirm the therapeutic effect of traction for reduction of a disc protrusion. However, long-term effects can only be obtained when the patient also performs the necessary prophylactic/self-treatment.

Sustained traction has three major effects on the lumbar spine:

- The distance between the vertebral bodies increases, which creates more space for reduction.

- The posterior longitudinal ligament tightens and thus exerts a centripetal force on the protrusion. This implies that a posterocentral protrusion will respond better to traction than will a posterolateral one.

- Discography shows that a subatmospheric pressure is induced, by means of which a centripetal force is exerted on the protrusion.

II. Indications

To reduce a disc protrusion/bulging/deformation, sustained traction yields better results than intermittent traction.

When using intermittent traction, make sure that the traction force during the "rest" phase is not less then 36 kilograms.

Sustained traction can be considered in the following disorders:

- A lumbar nuclear disc protrusion.

- A mixed protrusion (partly annular, partly nuclear).

- Patients describing S4 pain: only a very cautious attempt is advisable. In case of incontinence, the patient should be referred for further examination at once.

- An upper lumbar disc protrusion (L1 and L2).

- A recurrent disc protrusion at the same level after laminectomy.

- A primary posterolateral protrusion that has lasted less than 3 months.

- Every situation where decompression is advisable.

Remark—For the safety of both the patient and the therapist, those indications can only be diagnosed after careful clinical examination (i.e., a thorough interpretation of the patient's history and functional examination).

III. Contraindications

The following are contraindications for lumbar traction:

- Acute lumbago (annular or nuclear) (i.e., every situation where each movement causes twinges in the back and/or the lower limb is the contraindication): The patient might well be comfortable during the traction, but when the tension is released, he is much worse. It may be an hour or more before he can get off the traction table again. This should be avoided.

- An annular protrusion: If the patient has a "hard" protrusion (history: probably sudden onset of complaints), certain manipulation techniques are a better idea.

- Patients over 60-65 years of age: The water content of the disc has largely receded at that age, so the effect of traction will be minimal. Whether or not to apply traction in such cases is a subjective interpretation, depending on the information from the history. The oldest patient who received successful traction in my practice was 73 years old. This is, of course, an exception.

- Certain cases of sciatica:
    - With neurological deficit (sensory and/or motor);
    - With gross deviation sideways or in flexion;
    - Sciatica that has persisted for 6 months in a patient under 60 years of age.
- Primary posterolateral protrusion of over 3 months' duration.
- Pregnancy: from the fifth month onward.
- Respiratory or cardiac insufficiency (the patient cannot tolerate the tightness of the thoracic harness).
- A patient with a cold should not be put on traction because a cough or a sneeze during traction can be very painful. (The same is true for laughing!)
- Immediately after a manipulation session. When a manipulation session fails to bring about improvement, traction could be attempted the following day.
- Any situation in which traction cannot be given comfortably.

IV. Technique

A. Position of the Patient/Criteria

Traction can be given in several positions. The more common one is with the patient supine, using a pelvic and a thoracic harness with the straps positioned anteriorly. A small cushion is used under the patient's knees.

Photos 134 through 136

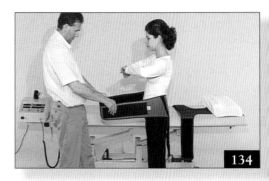

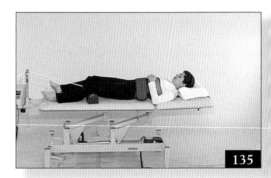

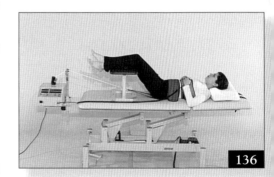

Some variations may be useful:

- If the patient is more comfortable in flexion (his extension in standing is probably painfully limited), a flexion bench under the patient's knees may increase comfort.

- If extension is comfortable, a small cushion can be used to support the lumbar spine.

Positions in prone lying are described in the literature that in theory seem useful; in practice, however, they are much less feasible and unneccesary.

Remark—It is more practical to put on the pelvic belt from a standing position.

B. Traction

Traction should preferably be sustained; a certain traction force should gradually be built in, maintained for some time, and then very slowly released (use the slowest release speed on the traction apparatus you use; go back to 0 kilogram in about 1 minute).

Sustained traction has a relaxing effect on muscle, and therefore the tension is transmitted to the joints themselves. After reaching the desired amount of traction, it takes some 3 minutes before electromyographic silence is obtained. This is one of the reasons why coninuous traction is preferred above intermittent traction. If you want to apply intermittent traction, make sure that the rest phase of the intermittent traction is not lower than 36 kilograms; In some cases, intermittent traction can optimize the subjective comfort of the patient.

1. Traction force

Opinions differ as to how many kilograms of traction force are needed. Levernieux found that a traction force of 10-30 kilograms results in a widening of about 1.5 millimeters between two lumbar vertebral bodies. Troisier obtained similar findings: a widening of 1 to 1.5 millimeters per level.

At least 30 to 35 kilograms are needed to have a beneficial effect in the lumbar spine (i.e., to reduce a disc protrusion). Others have demonstrated that the traction force should be at least 25% of the body weight. One study confirms that a traction force of less than 25% is equivalent to a placebo effect.

- The amount of traction used varies between 40 and 75 kilograms, depending on the patient's morphology and symptoms. We use the maximum traction force that is comfortable for the patient. The traction is held for some 30-45 minutes (most of the vertebral separation takes place in the first half hour). The traction for the first session is less: some 36 kilograms for about 20 minutes. In subsequent sessions, the duration and amount of traction increase.

- Treatment is best given on consecutive days. Two to three weeks are required.

- In each session, the patient is examined before applying traction to assess progress. Since the back can be tender for some minutes immediately after traction, the functional examination is done before applying traction to avoid a false positive interpretation. The articular movements in standing (extension and side flexions), trunk flexion with added neck flexion, and the SLR are the main control tests that can be used before traction.

2. After the traction

The tension should be released very gradually (choose the slowest possible release speed), without any abrupt movement. The harnesses are then opened, starting with the thoracic one. This should also be done smoothly to avoid painful twinges.

After traction, the patient should not stand up immediately. The evolution from decompression toward compression needs to happen gradually. The patient should perform some gentle movements in supine lying, flexing and extending a knee (note that the first movement could be a little bit difficult or even painful), then performing, with both knees flexed together, small pelvic rotations, and eventually lifting his pelvis off the table.

Photos 137 through 140

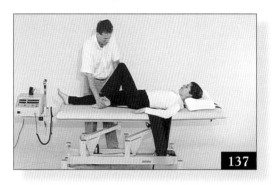

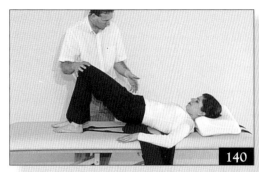

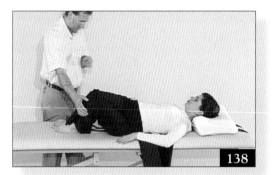

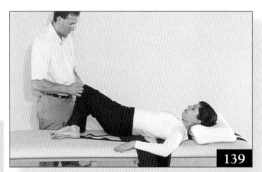

If the patient manages all this without discomfort, he can then get off the table. He should do so by rolling onto one side, bending both knees, bringing both feet outside the table, pushing himself up into a sitting position, and then standing up immediately.

Photo 141

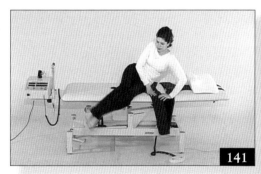

For the next 10 minutes or so, sitting should not be allowed; therefore, the patient should not remove his shoes before the treatment so as to avoid flexion postures afterward. Immediately after traction he should go for a little walk before driving home. He should drive as little as possible and only with a cushion behind the back; he should also avoid sitting as much as possible in the first half hour.

Remark—It is imperative that the patient respects his ADL advice after the traction, because the transition from decompression toward normal compression should evolve as favorably as possible.

V. Results

We expect improvement to start after a couple of days; if not, we should change the position in which traction is given (more flexion or extension?). If there is no improvement after 1 week, traction is abandoned.

About 2 to 3 weeks of traction (10-15 sessions) are normal. CT scan study shows reduction of disc material taking place in 78.5% of central, 66.6% of posterolateral, and 57.1% of lateral protrusions.

If the symptoms are much less after 2 weeks but have not disappeared completely, a third week's treatment follows.

VI. Prophylaxis After Traction or Manipulation

There are four elements in the active management of this type of problem:

- Reducing the derangement,
- Keeping it reduced,
- Recovery of function, and
- Prophylaxis.

Reduction of a disc protrusion is not sufficient. We have to minimize the chances of recurrence and help the patient to restore his function as soon as possible. The patient needs to be educated on the mechanisms that contribute to his symptoms, enhancing his understanding of why the treatment (including home exercises) is necessary to reduce symptoms and prevent recurrences. I specifically refer to McKenzie-related publications.

The patient should realize that certain postures and movements are favorable and others unfavorable. It is helpful to give him a leaflet/book on prophylaxis, with some advice on how to use his back. Experience shows, however, that patients do not immediately put these tips into practice. It takes a long time for patients to make lifestyle changes. The patient must first understand that a change needs to be made, and they must realize the benefit of making the change. It must also be reinforced that the lifestyle change must continue into pain-free episodes.

To make it even easier for the patient, I summarized some McKenzie principles on what I call the "Back Instruction Card."

Specific suggestions are made concerning lying down, sitting, standing up, changing postures, lifting weights, altering specific situations at work, and whether or not to practice sports activities.

Basically, three rules must be strictly respected:

- Keep your lumbar spine hollow.
- Change positions often.
- Flexion should be compensated by extension.

I. Indications

Most disc protrusions, except the nuclear self-reducing variant, can be manipulated.

II. Contraindications

Two absolute contraindications to manipulation are:

- The use of anticoagulant therapy and

- Spinal cord compression.

In the cervical spine chapter, we distinguish between minor compression (symptoms only) and more severe compression (symptoms and signs). Here, even a minor compression is an absolute contraindication.

Relative contraindication—No extension techniques in prone lying in elderly or osteoporotic patients for fear of a rib fracture.

III. Manipulation Techniques

In the cervical and lumbar spine, manipulations are totally nonspecific (there is no need for specificity). In the thoracic spine, we try to focus our manipulation on a certain level or levels. These techniques cannot really be called specific, but they are more focused. How can we find a "working level"? The way to do this is to use extension pressure on the spinous processes.

If pressure on one spinous process causes pain, we repeat the test on the spinous process just above and just below it. If either of these two is also painful, we have found a level.

In practice, it is also possible to get three positive answers (i.e., two affected levels).

At times, signs are so slight that an extension pressure is barely painful.

For central and unilateral manipulation techniques, the manipulating hand is placed on the lower vertebra of the specific level. For unilateral manipulation, we need to make contact with the transverse process instead of the spinous process. In the thoracic spine, the transverse processes are not level with the spinous processes. We have to look cephally for the transverse processes.

A. Location of the Transverse Processes

In relation to the spinous processes, the transverse processes are located one and a half levels up in the middle part (T4-T8/9), gradually less (one level, one-half level), more cranial and more caudal.

B. Manipulation Techniques

The manipulation technique for the thoracic spine begins with taking up the slack (bringing the body weight above the patient). Then, after asking the patient to relax, an assistant builds in traction, followed 1-2 seconds later by an extension manipulation. Reduction is obtained with strong traction and little manipulative strength. In the upper half of the thoracic spine, slightly more strength is used.

1. Positions for traction

- Traction on the arms for a protrusion between T6 and T12.

- Traction at the head for a protrusion above T6 or if the patient has a shoulder problem. The assistant makes sure to be in a position from which he can perform intensive traction. If a patient has specific shoulder complaints, then of course traction at the arms is out the question.

Remark—Never perform these manipulations without traction.

11

Photos 142 and 143

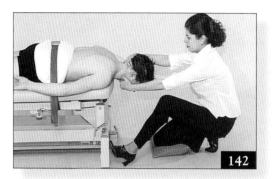

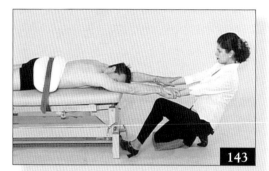

2. Manipulation: central extension pressure

Once the level has been found (see above), the middle of the therapist's fifth metacarpal bone is placed on the lower spinous process (e.g., level T8-T9: hand on T9). This hand is now brought more horizontal and reinforced by the other. The therapist leans against the table with his legs spread apart.

Execution—The therapist brings his body weight above the patient and takes up the slack. He then asks the patient to relax for a moment and orders, "Traction." The assistant pulls as hard as possible, and the manipulative thrust follows some 2 seconds later. (This small time lapse is needed to make sure that the traction becomes effective.)

The manipulation itself is a high-velocity, low-amplitude thrust toward extension, using the body weight with extended arms.

Photos 144 and 145

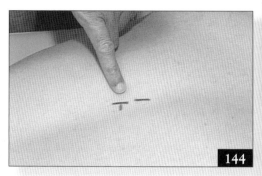

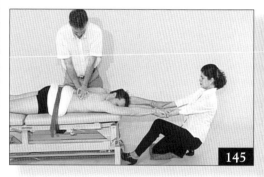

3. Manipulation: unilateral extension-rotation pressure

For a right rotation, the therapist stands at the patient's left side. He places the pisiform bone of the left or right hand on the right transverse process of the lower vertebra. For a bony contact, he first pulls the skin slightly toward himself and then pushes the paravertebral muscles aside. He reinforces the grip with the other hand, leans forward, and applies his body weight above his hands. Manipulation follows as in the previous technique.

Photo 146

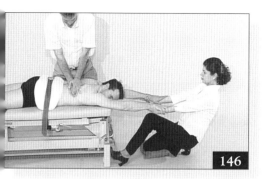

146

4. Manipulation: bilateral extension-rotation, "crossed" hands:

Grip—For a left rotation, the therapist stands at the patient's left side. He places his left pisiform bone on the left transverse process of the lower vertebra. Initially, his fingers point outward; then he turns his hand so that his fingers point downward. This allows him to move the muscles away from the spine so that he now has a bony contact on the transverse process. The trapezio-first metacarpal joint of the right hand is placed on the right transverse process of the upper vertebra in exactly the same way, first with the fingers pointing outward, then upward. The manipulation itself is performed just as in the previous technique.

Photos 147 through 149

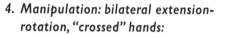

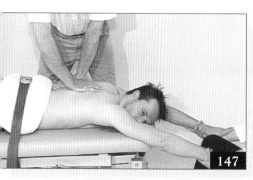

147

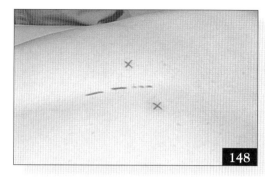

148

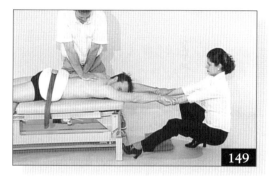

149

5. Manipulation: upper thoracic rotation

For a right rotation manipulation, the assistant should pull at the patient's head in some 10° of right rotation (for the patient's comfort). The therapist brings the patient's right shoulder backward with his left elbow and applies counterpressure with the other hand on the right half of the thorax, as high as possible. When the slack has been taken up, the patient has relaxed, and the order for traction has been given to the assistant, as in the previous techniques, manipulation is a swift trunk side flexion to the right under strong traction.

Photo 150

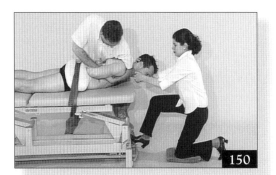

IV. Deep Friction Techniques

A. Deep Friction, Pectoralis Major

The DF is executed in the normal way with a pinching technique between the thumb and fingers. During the active phase, the therapist pulls the muscle fibers toward himself. He sits beside the table, which is set rather high; in this way, the DF can be given with the wrist in the neutral position.

Photo 151

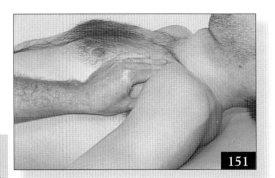

B. Deep Friction, Serratus Anterior

This structure becomes accessible by means of a medial rotation at the shoulder; if necessary, a cushion is placed under the patient's shoulder. In this way, the vertebral border of the scapula can easily be palpated.

The DF is executed in the normal way with the thumb flexed. The active phase is a pull downward, with pressure against the anterior aspect of the scapula.

Photo 152

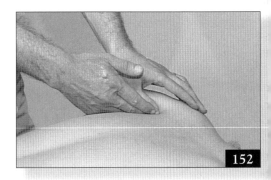

11

I. Introduction

The purpose of manipulation is reduction of a displaced fragment of disc. For obvious safety reasons, this needs to be done under (strong) traction. Traction also increases the efficiency. The same rules apply as in the lumbar spine: the first maneuver is always performed at half intensity, and we reassess after each maneuver (check the positive tests from the examination).

After taking up the slack, the manipulative thrust is given, but only if we feel a suitable end-feel. If a bone-to-bone end-feel or a muscle spasm are felt, we do not manipulate. The decision on whether or not to give the manipulative thrust is thus made at the end of the slack.

It is our firm conviction that the cervical manipulative techniques described below, if indicated, possess extraordinary inherent safety. We should realize that our aim is not to produce a "click"; a click can be heard but is certainly not the primary target. If our objective is the reduction of an internal derangement by manipulation, this can only be achieved safely by using sufficient longitudinal traction. This creates a negative pressure in the intervertebral joint, substantially reducing the risk of spinal cord compression.

Sometimes rotation or side flexion are added to this strong longitudinal traction. These articular movements are only guiding elements in our manipulation, changing biomechanical forces. A 100% complete rotation or side flexion beyond the articular and physiological limits is not necessary. Hence, we do not search for a position of maximal rotation or side flexion in which to manipulate. On the contrary, we remain largely within the physiological limits, which in the end substantially increases the safety of these techniques. Besides, the post-manipulative pain that often occurs when using specific "locking" techniques is significantly reduced or even absent. Another advantage is that the vertebral artery is subjected to less torsional influence if a manipulation is performed within the physiological limits.

It should be realized that many symptoms arising from the vertebral spine are negatively influenced by gravity. The Cyriax manipulative techniques partially and temporarily neutralize this negative influence of gravity. In this way, we can obtain a better therapeutic result with less risk.

When checking the positive tests of the clinical examination after the first manipulation, what is considered an improvement?

- Less pain,

- More mobility,

- Fewer painful movements,

- Shortening of the pain, and

- The appearance of a painful arc.

Be sure to assess the correct pain and not transient post-manipulative soreness.

II. Indications

A. Disc Protrusions

- *Acute torticollis*—In patients under 30 years of age, a special procedure is needed, which will be discussed later.

- *Unilateral cervicoscapular aching*—In 90% of cases, three or four sessions are enough to achieve a reduction.

- *Unilateral root pain*—Bear in mind that we expect this clinical pattern only in patients over 35. The protrusion is considered irreducible in the second half of its spontaneous recovery and in case of neurological deficit (motor and/or sensory—see Part I.)

- *Central protrusion*—Here, only techniques with a maximum of traction and a minimum of articular movement are used (i.e., a strong, straight pull and no rotation techniques). There is a real risk of spinal cord compression if these rules are not adhered to.

- *Bilateral protrusion*—The same techniques are used as for a central protrusion. The prognosis, though, is not favorable.

The following scheme gives an overview of some clinical images and the chances of reducibility.

Reducibility of cervical disc protrusions	Reducible
1. Scapular pain, no root pain, no neurological deficit	1-2 sessions
2. Unilateral scapular pain with root pain, favorable neck signs, no neurological deficit	almost certainly
3. Unilateral scapular pain with root pain, unfavorable neck signs, no neurological deficit	not?
4. Slight bilateral arm ache, paresthesia in hands and/or feet, good neck signs, no deficit	50% in 1-4 sessions
5. Unilateral root pain with distal onset and proximal evolution	not
6. Unilateral scapular pain with root pain, minor paresthesia, good neck signs, root pain less than 1 month	sometimes
7. Unilateral scapular pain with root pain, neurological deficit	not
8. Unilateral scapular pain with root pain and a recovering deficit; root pain of more than 6 months' standing, good neck signs (the first manipulation session abolishes the scapular ache and restarts the mechanism of spontaneous recovery; a few days later, the root pain begins to ease); two to three manipulation sessions at intervals of 2 weeks	2-3 sessions
9. Unilateral scapular pain persisting for months after a root pain has ceased; only one neck movement is painful	not
10. Paresthesia in hands and/or feet, evoked by neck flexion; no spastic gait, negative plantar reflex	yes?
11. Swift evolution: scapular pain, the next day root pain and paresthesia, good neck signs, no deficit yet	very seldom
12. Elastic recoil; one expects an easy reduction by manipulation. A full-range rotation manipulation is possible but a rubbery rebound is felt at the end of range; on assessing the result afterward, the limitation remains unaltered. This rare nuclear protrusion needs sustained traction in bed.	not
13. Paresthesia in hands and/or feet, positive Babinski	not

B. Other Disorders

- *Basilar vertigo*—Cervicogenic vertigo is a moderate indication for manipulation. Only straight pull is used.

- *Migraine*—Manipulation is successful in some 10-20% of cases, particularly in patients over 40. The techniques used are rotation and side flexion under strong traction. A beginning attack can sometimes be stopped with 30 seconds of strong traction. This has been discovered purely by coincidence; the mechanism remains unclear.

- *Tinnitus*—The rate of success is slightly less than for migraine. The same techniques as for vertigo are used.

- *Capsuloligamentous pain with or without limitation of movement*—

  – Cervical pain or headache.

  – Two manipulative techniques: rotation and side flexion.

  – Two ways of manipulating:

    -- A "quick stretch" for rupturing adhesions

      - In case of diffuse capsular adhesions after an injury or

      - In cases of early osteoarthrosis.

    -- A "slow stretch" (capsular stretching) for:

      - Advanced osteoarthrosis,

      - Ankylosing spondylitis,

      - "The old man's matutinal headache,"

      - Facet joint arthrosis.

    -- Two absolute contraindications for using these techniques are:

  - A disc protrusion and

  - Basilar ischemia.

III. Contraindications

A. Absolute Contraindications

- *Pressure on the spinal cord*—The presence of symptoms (extrasegmental paresthesia) without signs (negative Babinski):

  – A careful attempt (only straight pull) for reduction is still possible.

  – Symptoms with signs: an absolute bar for manipulation.

- *Basilar ischemia*—Straight pull technique can be used.

- *Drop-attacks*—Occlusion of both vertebral arteries on hyperextension, with the patient falling to the ground without losing consciousness. There is a congenital upper cervical abnormity: hypertrophy of the odontoid process, with ligamentous laxity.

- *Rheumatoid arthritis*—Ligamentous laxity: a danger of subluxation and consequent contusion of the spinal cord on manipulation.

- Anticoagulants—Danger of an intraspinal hematoma causing spinal cord compression. This is a contraindication in the entire vertebral spine. If manipulation is advisable, the medical doctor can decide to suspend the anticoagulant therapy for a while.

- *Dural adherences* (at the vertebral body or the PLL)—Extrasegmental paresthesia (hands and feet) at taking up the slack (i.e., at building in the traction) or during neck flexion. This is very rare.

Cervical Manipulation and Deep Friction

12

B. Relative Contraindications

- *Central protrusion*—No rotation techniques can be used; only techniques with a longitudinal traction component and side flexion techniques are indicated.

- *Acute torticollis in patients under 30*—Special "Bateman's" procedure (see IV).

- *Gross deformity*—This suggests a large protrusion, which makes the reduction more difficult. Concentrate on the deformity first; build in traction in the direction of the deviation.

- *The appearance of arm pain*—Any technique that produces or worsens arm pain should be abandoned.

C. Cases When Manipulation Is Useless

- *There is no protrusion at the moment.*

- *Root pain*—

  - In the second half of the spontaneous evolution (see Part I).

  - If there is neurological deficit (motor or sensory).

  - PPLP.

  - Swift progression: onset of scapular pain one day, followed by root pain and paresthesia the next day.

- *Root pain with unfavorable neck signs*—A neck movement that produces/worsens pain down the arm is an unfavorable sign for manipulation.

- *Nuclear protrusion*—The patient is probably young. There are two particular findings when attempting manipulation:

  - Full rotation is achieved during manipulation/traction; assessment afterward shows that the limitation is unaltered.

  - An unsuitable end-feel (elastic recoil) on manipulation.

Remark—It has been suggested that deep friction of the splenius and semispinalis capitis muscles could help to get better relaxation. I believe that relaxation is obtained more easily by involving your patient—by explaining the pathology and the purpose of what you are doing.

IV. Special Strategy for Acute Torticollis in Patients Under 30

Because the protrusion probably has a more nuclear character, this particular strategy is used in the first treatment session:

1. Straight pull in the line of the deviation.

2. Manipulation in the free direction:

   - Rotation,

   - Side flexion.

3. Bateman's procedure in the limited direction:

   - Rotation,

   - Side flexion.

The patient lies supine. The head is brought passively into the painful rotation. After only a few gradations, pain appears; this posture is maintained until the pain eases (and/or centralizes). We then go a little farther in the limited direction until a new pain appears, wait until it eases, and so on.

It might take from a half hour to an hour for full rotation to be reached. The neck is then brought back to neutral by a rather quick movement under slight traction; during this movement, a twinge can be felt. The same gradual positioning of the neck into the limited range of side flexion then follows. Since the protrusion has already been largely reduced, this should take no more than 10 minutes.

The entire first session lasts perhaps an hour and a half, but the patient is 90% better.

So as not to lose the benefit of the treatment, a last element is important:

4. Advice—The patient should repeat the Bateman's actively at home, and he should try to sleep at night with his head well supported in lordosis. Various types of orthopaedic cushions can be helpful.

In the second treatment session, we continue with the normal strategy.

Remark—Take your time in performing this strategy; being in a hurry has unfavorable results.

V. Techniques

A. Slow Stretch, Rotation

For a rotation to the right, the therapist's right hand grasps the patient's chin in pronation; the therapist then steps slightly backward with his right foot to build in some traction. We reach the end of range, stretch, and remain in this position for up to 1 minute.

Photo 153

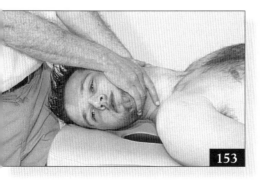

B. Slow Stretch, Side Flexion

One hand, placed laterally in the lower cervical spine, acts as a fulcrum. The other hand, placed on the temporal bone, brings the neck into side flexion and eventually stretches the capsule.

The lower cervical fulcrum is important for reaching the articular end of range and to avoid creating too much tension on the trapezius muscle.

Photo 154

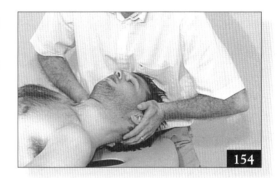

C. Quick Stretch, Rotation

We use the same grip as for the slow stretch. This time, there is hardly any traction. A swift rotation thrust is used at the end of range.

Important—High velocity, low amplitude.

Photo 155

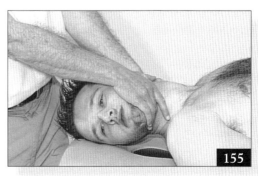

Cervical Manipulation and Deep Friction

12

D. Quick Stretch, Side Flexion

Agalin, we use the same grip as for the slow stretch. A swift "shearing" thrust with both hands is used at the end of range.

Photo 156

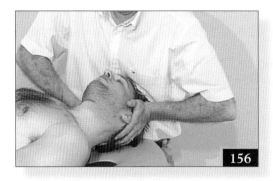

E. Deep Friction, Facet Joint

This DF can be done with the patient sitting or lying prone (I prefer the sitting position). As we palpate from the occiput downward, the first bone we feel is the spinous process of C2. Between the spinous processes of C2 and C3, we move forward and find the facet joint on a vertical line from the mastoid process.

The DF is as follows: We use a flat thumb to take a reserve of skin in an upward and slightly anterior direction; pressure is then applied. The active phase is a downward-posterior movement. It is an arm movement in which the elbow moves upward as the thumb moves downward (a sort of half-moon movement), and vice versa. The other hand stabilizes the patient's head.

Photo 157

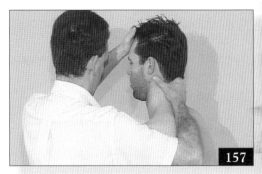

F. Manipulation: Straight Pull

The patient lies supine with the shoulders against the shoulder support and the head beyond the edge of the table. If no shoulder support is available, an assistant holds both legs and the head does not have to be brought beyond the edge of the table.

One of the therapist's hands grasps the occiput and the other hand is hooked under the patient's chin. The therapist avoids pinching with his fingers.

The correct sequence of the manipulation is as follows: right hand at the occiput, right foot against the leg of the table (toes pointing to the left), left hand at the patient's chin, left foot against the leg of the table (toes pointing to the left). The therapist's knees are well bent and the arms straight (in order to build in traction with the body weight); both hands now perform a quick manipulative thrust in a longitudinal direction, after which the therapist takes a small step backward with one foot in order to gradually release the traction.

Photos 158 through 160

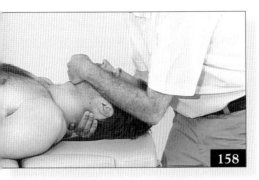

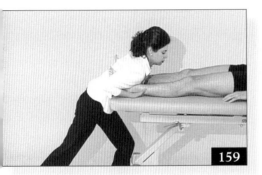

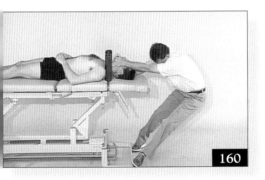

If no assistant is available, the patient can grasp the table in order to fix himself.

Photo 161

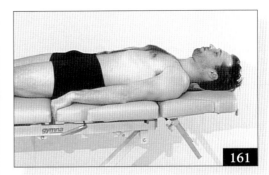

Remark—The therapist should avoid building in flexion, thus pulling himself up by using the patient's head.

G. Manipulation: Traction-Rotation

The patient's posture is the same as in the previous technique. For a full rotation manipulation, the patient's head should be beyond the edge of the table.

Grip—For a rotation to the left, the therapist's left hand is placed at the chin and his feet point to the left.

The sequence for a half rotation to the left is: right hand at the occiput, right foot against the table, left hand at the chin, left foot against the table, knee flexion, arm extension, build in a half rotation, followed by a quick and short rotation thrust; bring the head back to the neutral position and release the traction by taking a small step backward.

The full rotation technique differs from that of half rotation in that the main part of taking up the slack is now obtained using a trunk side flexion; after assessing the end-feel, a quick manipulative thrust is given with both hands.

Remark—Both a hard and a spastic end-feel indicate that the manipulative thrust should not be given.

Cervical Manipulation and Deep Friction

12

Photos 162 and 163

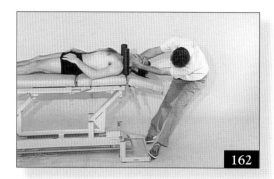

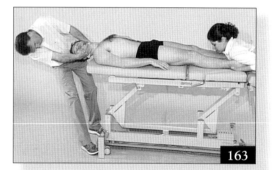

H. Manipulation: Side Flexion

The starting position for a side flexion to the left is with the patient lying on the left half of the table, his shoulders level and his head beyond the edge of the table. The assistant immobilizes the patient's right shoulder; his left foot is braced against the leg of the table.

Grip—The therapist's left hand is placed on the occiput; the MCP joint of his index finger lies between two spinous processes. The therapist now moves his hand sideways, keeping the thumb in extension to avoid putting pressure anteriorly on the neck. The little finger maintains the patient's head in a midposition and avoids extension.

Execution—The therapist's left foot is more or less under the left shoulder of the patient. He bends his knee, bringing his right leg far backward, and stretches his arms as far as possible to build in enough traction. The neck is then brought into side flexion and a swift manipulative thrust follows; the manipulation is an adduction at the right shoulder.

Remark—It is important for the left hand, placed laterally on the spine, to act as a fulcrum for the side flexion. If this hand moves toward the left, the manipulation becomes impossible and too much tension is created on the trapezius muscle.

Hint—Bend the left knee a bit more and move anteriorly with your body weight; this makes it easier to keep your left hand steady.

Photos 164 through 166

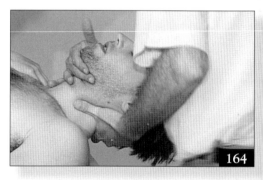

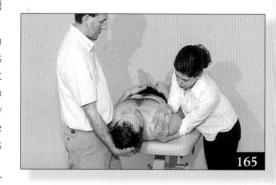

12

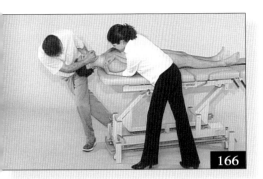

166

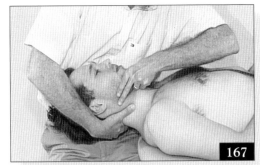

167

I. Manipulation: Anterior Glide

The patient's head hangs over the edge of the table. His shoulders are immobilized by shoulder supports or by an assistant positioned at the legs.

Grip—One of the therapist's hands is placed on the chin, with ring and little fingers bent under it for applying traction. The other hand cradles the occiput.

Execution—The therapist is positioned with his right hand at the occiput, his left foot against the table, his left hand at the chin, and his right foot against the table. By moving the right foot forward, the therapist now hangs at the patient's head, thus creating sufficient traction. It is important for the therapist to support the patient's head with his abdomen. The patient's head and the therapist's abdomen and hands form one entity.

The manipulation then consists of a knee flexion, thus creating an anteroposterior gliding movement.

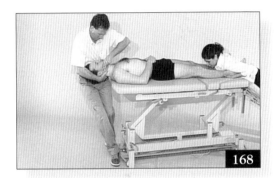

168

J. Manipulation: Side Glide

The patient's lies supine with the head over the edge of the table. An assistant immobilizes the patient's thorax at the elbow and shoulder, at the same time using his abdomen as another fulcrum of stability. The therapist grasps the patient's head with both hands and uses his abdomen as a cushion for the head. The fingers are placed on the occiput, and both thenars lie well forward.

The maneuver is not a proper manipulation; it is more a mobilization consisting of repeated side gliding movements. Again, the patient's head and the therapist's hands and abdomen form one entity. The side gliding is obtained by shifting the body weight laterally.

Cervical Manipulation and Deep Friction

12

Photo 169

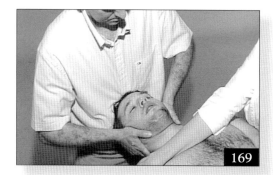

169

VI. Manipulative Strategy

A. Unilateral Protrusion (1)

For a successful treatment by manipulation, the patient should be confident and should understand the nature of his problem. Under these circumstances, the "green evolution" (explained below) seems to be the best procedure in most cases. Assessment shows an improvement after each maneuver.

The normal sequence is as follows:

- In the most comfortable direction (the rotation direction in which the patient moves best), we first perform a one-half rotation, assess, then a three-quarter rotation, assess, and finally a full rotation manipulation.

- We can do the same in the other direction: one-half ⇒ three-quarters ⇒ full rotation.

- If necessary, the side flexion technique is performed (1-3x) in only one direction: away from the painful side.

The session ends with the lateral glide technique to remove any new soreness that may have developed due to the maneuvers. The patient returns 1-2 days later for the next session. (As with the lumbar spine: for elderly patients, fewer manipulations in one session and a longer interval between the sessions.)

Remark—If the symptoms are significantly improved at the end of the session but extension has not improved much, an AP glide may be useful. This maneuver improves extension, in particular. It is not always necessary to perform this strategy in its totality; sometimes two to three maneuvers will suffice

B. Unilateral Protrusion (2)

Now we discuss the situation in which a maneuver either has left the patient unchanged or has made him worse. Remember one of the fundamental rules: Never increase the intensity of a maneuver when its low-intensity version has not improved the patient.

1. Track 1

The point of departure is, as always, a half rotation in the comfortable direction; following that, the patient seems to be unchanged:

- An unchanged condition means this rotation is not suited to the patient; manipulation under traction can be continued, but try another maneuver.

Two further techniques can be tried next at low intensity: rotation in the opposite direction and side flexion away from the painful side.

A maneuver that helps is repeated; one that does not help is abandoned.

2. Track 2

After the half rotation in the comfortable direction, the patient is worse. A logical step backward is needed, such as a straight pull. The result of this second technique can be:

- *Worse:* After two techniques with unfavorable results, manipulation is abandoned. Reassess.

- *Better:* Repeat the straight pull as long as it helps. Then go back to the starting point, and hopefully the "green evolution" will be reached again. It may then be advisable to start with a one-quarter rotation. Reassess.

- *Unchanged:* Manipulation under traction can continue; the first rotation was not suited to this patient. Two further possibilities remain: side flexion away from the painful side and the other rotation, both at low intensity.

If a maneuver helps, it is repeated, after which the therapist comes back to the starting point. If the patient is worse again, manipulation is abandoned.

C. Central Protrusion

A central disc protrusion constitutes an increased danger of spinal cord compression during manipulation. Rotation techniques, as well as manipulation techniques without sufficient traction, are absolutely contraindicated.

This time, the starting point is the straight pull; this maneuver should be repeated four to five times, gradually increasing the intensity.

As for the second technique, a choice is possible:

- We can use the side flexion technique (the difference compared with a unilateral protrusion is that here one can open in both directions; therefore, the side flexion technique will be used bilaterally) or

- We can use an AP glide, but this can only be used when the protrusion has largely reduced (because we have less traction than in the other techniques).

When one method proves unsuccessful, it is always possible to change to the other method.

Related Reading List

Bijl, D., et al. (1998). "Validity of Cyriax's concept capsular pattern for the diagnosis of osteoarthritis of hip and/or knee," *Scand J Rheumatol*, 27(5): 347-51.

Bowling, R.W., et al. (1994). "Cyriax reexamined," *Phys Ther*, 74(11): 1073-5.

Broccard, J. (1996). "L'approche Cyriax de l'épicondylite," *Physiotherapie*, Jg 32, nr 12: 9-10.

Brosseau, L., et al. (2002). "Deep transverse friction massage for treating tendinitis," *Cochrane Database Syst Rev*, (1): CD003528.

Butler, D. (2000). "The sensitive nervous system," Noigroup Publications, Australia.

Chamberlain, G. (1982). "Cyriax's friction massage: A review," *J Orthop Sport Phys Therap*, Summer.

Chesworth, B.M., et al. (1998). "Movement diagram and "end-feel" reliability when measuring passive lateral rotation of the shoulder in patients with shoulder pathology," *Phys Ther*, 78(6): 593-601.

Claeys, Jan, et al. (2000), *Orthopedische Geneeskunde Cyriax in theorie en praktijk, deel II: behandeling d.m.v. infiltratie en injectie*, SATAS.

Cyriax, J.H. (1982). *Textbook of Orthopaedic Medicine, Volume I: Diagnosis of Soft Tissue Lesions*, 8th edition; Ballière Tindall.

Cyriax, J.H., (1980). *Textbook of Orthopaedic Medicine, Volume II: Treatment by Manipulation, Massage and Injection*, 10th edition; Ballière Tindall.

Cyriax, J.H. (1980). "Manipulation trials," *Br Med J*, 280(6207): 111.

Cyriax, J.H. (1978). "Dural pain," *Lancet*, 1(8070): 919-21.

Cyriax, J.H. (1977) "Deep massage," *Physiother*, 63(2): 60-1

De Coninck, Steven, and Meeus, Kurt (2003). Relevantie van het klinisch onderzoek met betrekking tot de diagnosestelling van een supraspinatus tendinitis, Thesis KHBO, June.

De Coninck, Steven (2000). "Klinische Untersuchung der Schulter: sprechen Therapeuten die gleiche Sprache?" *Krankengymnastik - Zeitschrift für Physiotherapeuten*, Jg 52, nr 8, Seiten 1358-136; Cyriax Assessment Form®.

De Coninck, Steven, et al. (1999). *Orthopedische Geneeskunde Cyriax in theorie en praktijk, deel I: onderzoek en diagnose*, SATAS.

De Coninck, Steven, et al. (1999). *Orthopedische Geneeskunde Cyriax in theorie en praktijk, deel II: behandeling d.m.v. diepe dwarse frictie, manipulatie en tractie*, SATAS.

Donatelli, R., and Owen-Burhkardt, H. (1984). "Effects of immobilization on the extensibility of periarticular connective tissue," *J Orthop Sport Phys Therap*, 3, 2.: 67-72.

Ellis, R.M. (1995). "Cyriax's passive motion tests," *Phys Ther*, 75(3): 239-40.

Evans, Ph. (1980). "The healing process at cellular level: A review," *Physiother*, 66(8): 256-9.

Flock, Henrik (2000). "Der Freie Gelenkkörper im arthrotishen Gelenk," *Krankengymnastik - Zeitschrift für Physiotherapeuten*, Jg 52, nr 9, Seiten 1474-1482.

Franklin, M.F., et al. (1996). "Assessment of exercise-induced minor muscle lesions: The accuracy of Cyriax's diagnosis by selective tension paradigm," *J Orthop Sports Phys Ther*, 24(3): 122(9).

Fritz, J.M., et al. (1998). "An examination of the selective tissue tension scheme with evidence for the concept of a capsular pattern of the knee," *Phys Therap*, 78(10): 1046-56.

Gould, A. (1995). "Manual therapy for a prolapsed intervertebral disc: A critical evaluation of two approaches," *British Journal of Therapy and Rehabilitation,* 2(12): 663-668.

Greenwood, M.J., et al. (1998). "Differential diagnosis of the hip versus lumbar spine: five case reports," *J Orthop sports Phys Ther,* 27(4): 308-15.

Hayes, K.W., et al. (1994). "An examination of Cyriax's passive motion test with patients having osteoarthritis of the knee," *Phys Ther,* 74(8): 697-707.

Kesson, M., et al. (1998). *Orthopaedic Medicine, A Practical Approach:* Butterworth-Heinemann.

Krause, M., et al (2000). "Lumbar spine traction: Evaluation of effects and recommended application for treatment," *Manual Therapy,* 5(2): 72-81.

Laslett, M. (1996). *Mechanical Diagnosis and Therapy: The Upper Limb.* Minneapolis, MN: Occupational Physical Therapy Products.

McKenzie, R.A. (1992). *The Lumbar Spine, Mechanical Diagnosis and Therapy:* Spinal Publications Limited, New Zealand.

McKenzie, R.A., (2000). *The Cervical and Thoracic Spine, Mechanical Diagnosis and Therapy:* Spinal Publications Limited, New Zealand.

McKenzie, R.A., and May, Stephen (1995). *The Human Extremities, Mechanical Diagnosis and Therapy:* Spinal Publications Limited, New Zealand.

Mehne, S. (1996). "Systematische Physiotherapie bei Bandscheibenvorfall," *Krankengymnastik,* Jg 48, nr 6:. 838-846, 863-869.

Ombregt, L., et al. (1995). *A System of Orthopaedic Medicine:* Saunders.

Ombregt, L. (2000). "Het durale concept," *Kine,* 93(5): 17-20.

Pellecchia, G.L., et al. (1996). "Intertester reliability of the Cyriax evaluation in assessing patients with shoulder pain," *J Orthop Sports Phys Ther,* 23(1): 34-8.

Petersen, Ch. M., et al. (2000). "Construct validity of Cyriax's selective tension examination: Association of end-feels with pain at the knee and shoulder," *J Orthop Sports Phys Ther,* 30(9) 512-527.

Ridulfo, Giuseppe, and Festa Nicola (2000). "Accordo diagnostico nella valutazione della spalla secondo Cyriax con le Cyriax Assessment Forms," *Terapia Manuale & Riabilitazione,* 2.4: 35-38.

Sachse, J. (1996). "Zum Kapselmuster des Schultergelenkes," *Man Med,* Jg 34, nr 6: 86-87

Schwellnus, M.P., et al. (1992). "Deep transverse frictions in the treatment of the iliotibial band friction syndrome in athletes: A clinical trial,' *Physiotherapy,* 78(8): 564-8.

Troisier, O. (1991). "Tennis elbow," *Rev Prat,* 41(18): 1651-5.

van der Wurff, P., et al. (2000). "Clinical tests of the sacroiliac joint; A systematic methodologica review. Part 2: Validity," *Manual Therapy,* 5(2) 89-96.

Verhaar, J.A. (1994). "Tennis elbow: Anatomical epidemiological and therapeutic aspects," *Int orthop,* 18(5): 263-7.

Verhaar, J.A. (1996). "Local corticosteroid injection versus Cyriax-type physiotherapy for tennis elbow," *J Bone Joint Surg Br,* 78(1): 128-32.

Vorselaars, J. (1991). "Hoe effectief zijn dwarse fricties bij bandletsels?" *Respons,* Jg 2 nr 12.

Waskowitz, R.S., et al. (1996). "Local corticosteroid injection versus Cyriax-type physiotherapy for tennis elbow," *Clin J Sport Med,* 6(4) 276.

Woodman, R.M., and Pare, L. (1982). "Evaluation and treatment of soft tissue lesions of the ankle and forefoot using the Cyriax approach: A case report," *Phys Ther*, 62(8): 1144-7.

Zimny, N.J. (1998). "Clinical reasoning in the evaluation and management of undiagnosed chronic hip pain in a young adult," *Phys Ther*, 78(1): 62-73.

Related Reading List

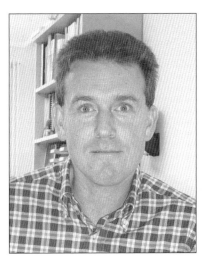

Steven L.H. De Coninck

"Steven L.H. De Coninck, MSc PT, is a senior teacher of the European Teaching Group of Orthopaedic Medicine Cyriax (ETGOM) and presents OMCyriax courses all over the world. He has a private practice in De Haan, Belgium, and published already several books, video productions and created the standardized Cyriax Assessment Forms.

Constantly innovating, updating and spreading the real basic value of OMCyriax is his mission. For more information go to www.etgom.be

The author can be contacted through info@etgom.be.